healing journeys

healing journeys

The Power of Rubenfeld Synergy

EDITED BY

Vicki Mechner

OmniQuest Press

CHAPPAQUA, NEW YORK

Published by OmniQuest Press

Book design by Cindy LaBreacht   Cover design by Sharon Lee Ryder

Publisher's Cataloging-in-Publication *(Provided by Quality Books, Inc.)*

Healing journeys : the power of Rubenfeld Synergy / edited by Vicki Mechner ; [foreword by Ilana Rubenfeld]. —1st ed.
    p. cm.
    Includes bibliographical references and index.
    Preassigned LCCN: 98-67158
    ISBN: 0–96642–613–4 (alk. paper)

    1. Mind and body therapies—Case studies.   2. Psychotherapy—Popular works.   3. Touch—Therapeutic use.   4. Healing.   I. Mechner, Vicki.

RC489.M53M43 1998   615.89   QBI98–66790
10 9 8 7 6 5 4 3 2 1
Printed in the United States of America.
First printing.

To my parents,
Oscar and Mary Weitzberg,
who taught me by their example:
Dad, that I have something to learn
from every person I meet, and
Mom, that I can accomplish anything
if I set my mind to it.

Contents

vii

healing journeys

contents

contents

Appendices

Foreword

Ilana Rubenfeld

In the early sixties I explored, researched, and developed an integration of bodywork and psychotherapy into a dynamic and holistic healing system, which I later named the Rubenfeld Synergy Method. It took many years for the pieces of the puzzle to fit into place, and when they did I began to practice and demonstrate this method and its healing power.

The simultaneous use of talk and listening touch was particularly exciting. Each was a powerful tool on its own, but together they enabled clients to journey deeper and integrate emotions and insights on a cellular level. Increasing numbers of people asked for Rubenfeld Synergy sessions. Not able to accommodate them, I began to consider training others.

In 1977 a group of bodyworkers, psychotherapists, counselors, artists, and musicians asked me to train them to be Rubenfeld Synergists. It's one thing to practice Rubenfeld Synergy with individuals and groups. It's quite another to develop ways to teach the method's philosophy, essence, and techniques to other people. The prospect challenged me, and I couldn't resist. I was determined to pass the method on.

Looking back, I appreciate how my studies as a conductor at the Juilliard School of Music prepared me for training others. To conduct music you must be able to follow ten to thirty parts simultaneously—while moving your body, expressing yourself in a nonverbal way, and touching the heart and spirit of the music. Conductors learn to do this by analyzing the music—taking it apart voice by voice—and then reintegrating it while remembering the sound and form of the whole composition. This way of learning was an ideal foundation for training future Synergists.

During the first training program, I played all the "instruments"—therapist, supervisor, administrator, and advisor, as well as curriculum developer. In the twenty-one years since then, the teaching faculty has grown substantially, and the training program has expanded to four years.

People who take the Rubenfeld Synergy Training Program come to it from various backgrounds. Some have been trained as psychotherapists, social workers, counselors, psychologists, and expressive arts therapists. Others have been educated as physicians, nurses, osteopaths, chiropractors, physical therapists, massage therapists, and practitioners of other types of bodywork. Still others are musicians and other performing artists, writers, visual artists, producers, businesspeople, and so on.

Everyone brings to the training a unique background and life story and particular ways of observing and experiencing the world.

As these multifaceted individuals share their different perspectives and vantage points during the training, they enrich each other's understanding of what they see, hear, and feel, and they come to understand their own prior knowledge and skills in a broader context.

In my forthcoming book, *The Listening Hand*, I will share a detailed history and philosophy of Rubenfeld Synergy, descriptions of sessions, and instructions for exercises that readers can do on their own. *Healing Journeys* is a magnificent overture to *The Listening Hand*. Some major themes that run through the stories in *Healing Journeys* are compassion, pain, curiosity, grief, humor, betrayal, and profound personal changes. The stories reflect a wide variety of perspectives.

I wish to acknowledge Vicki Mechner, editor of *Healing Journeys* and a graduate of the eleventh training class, for playing midwife extraordinaire to these stories. Some of the contributing writers told me how patiently she guided, cajoled, questioned, and supported them in expressing their experiences so that you, the reader, could share in the miracles that are possible through Rubenfeld Synergy.

I am moved to read how my students have taken my work with such integrity and care and expressed it through their own personal styles. They exemplify the philosophy and feeling behind the Rubenfeld Synergy logo—hands surrounding a heart, symbolizing the healing touch that comes from a heartfelt place of caring and compassion.

It is with pride and joy that I invite you to relish these stories and allow them to inspire you.

Ilana Rubenfeld
New York City
Summer 1998

ABOUT ILANA RUBENFELD

Ilana Rubenfeld is a world-recognized pioneer in integrating psychotherapy, intuition, and bodywork. Ilana directs bodymind energy as if she were conducting a symphony—and well she should. She graduated from the Juilliard School of Music and enjoyed a career in music conducting until a debilitating back spasm redirected her life journey toward healing and teaching.

Since her development of the Rubenfeld Synergy Method in the 1960s, Ilana has been a frequent presenter at conferences around the world. She is in demand as a keynote speaker and workshop leader—not only for the wisdom she imparts, but also because of her talents as a humorist and icebreaker.

Ilana is a faculty member of the Omega and Esalen Institutes and the New York Open Center. In 1994 she received the Association of Humanistic Psychology's Pathfinder Award for outstanding and innovative contributions to the field of humanistic psychology. In 1998 the International University of Professional Studies awarded Ilana an honorary doctorate in transpersonal psychology. She is currently writing The Listening Hand *for Bantam Books.*

Introduction

Vicki Mechner

"**What is** Rubenfeld Synergy?" Ever since my first session I have searched for a simple way to convey the essence of this subtle, multifaceted approach to healing. It is difficult to explain how its few simple elements—touch, talk, imagination, and humor—can promote healing. The brilliance of the work lies in the way these elements can be adapted to each client's situation, helping Synergist[1] and client tap into the wisdom of the body and explore how profoundly it is connected to the mind and emotions.

The idea for a collaborative book about Rubenfeld Synergy came to me several months after my certification. When I wrote to my fellow Synergists asking for submissions, more than sixty

---

[1] "Certified Rubenfeld Synergist" is the title used by certified practitioners.

responded with proposals and drafts. I decided to include only the personal and anecdotal stories because they seemed to convey the essence of the Rubenfeld Synergy Method better than the essays. Varying greatly in content and style, the stories illuminate different aspects of the method. Together they form a mosaic that reveals the big picture.

Some early readers of *Healing Journeys* asked questions that are not addressed directly in any of the stories. Here they are.

"Why do Synergists say 'client' instead of 'patient'?" "Patient" connotes passive treatment, and Rubenfeld Synergy requires clients' active participation. Where "patient" implies that a therapy or therapist may be able to *cure* from the outside, Rubenfeld Synergy supports a process of *healing* from within. Although the Synergist plays a major role in this process, it is the client who is responsible for change.

"Are Synergists qualified to deal with serious mental or physical illness?" Although the Rubenfeld Synergy Method does not diagnose or treat specific conditions, Synergists are trained to recognize situations in which referral for medical or psychiatric care is appropriate.

"Are all sessions as dramatic as the ones in the stories?" No. The authors chose to write about experiences that were particularly meaningful to them. In an effort to keep their stories short and engaging, they focused on highlights of their personal journeys.

"Do the results last beyond the session?" This depends on a client's ability and commitment to integrate new awareness into daily life. Most people need additional sessions to help them recognize old habits in new disguises, and to incorporate fledgling attitudes and behavior into their real-life situations and relationships.

"Does a person need to have previous experience with counseling or psychotherapy in order to benefit from Rubenfeld Synergy?" No. A few of the writers had no experience with therapy before trying Rubenfeld Synergy. Almost everyone can find sources of healing within. Let me give you an example.

*When Tom,** an old friend of the family, stays with us he sometimes does the grocery shopping. Having grown up in farm country, Tom really knows his fruits and vegetables. He also knows we love avocados, especially the sweet, nutty ones. One day Tom brought home some avocados that were heavily scarred. Curious, I asked why he had chosen them.

"Fruits with scars taste sweeter," he answered.

After thinking about that for a moment I said, half to myself, "Just like people," and turned to do some kitchen chores while Tom put away the groceries.

A few minutes later he said, "I agree. People without problems don't have as much character as people who have suffered." Then he told me about chronic pain from an old neck and shoulder injury, which he feared would never fully heal.

"But when I see a piece of scarred fruit," Tom explained, "it gives me hope. I figure that if the fruit could heal, so can I."

Our conversation had some of the earmarks of Rubenfeld Synergy sessions—trust, conversation that flows without being directing toward a particular outcome, and the exploration of feelings through the use of metaphor. In Rubenfeld Synergy sessions, metaphors often emerge and develop through the use of touch.

---

* This is not his real name. Throughout the book, asterisks are used to indicate names that have been changed to protect individuals' privacy. Identifying details are changed as well.

Touch was not an element of my conversation with Tom, but metaphor was: Tom had developed his own.

Healing often occurs in unexpected ways. I hope that some of the stories in *Healing Journeys* speak to you and serve you on your journey to self-discovery and healing.

Confidentiality

The stories in this book are based on actual situations the authors have encountered. Wherever possible the authors have contacted the individuals involved and obtained permission to use their stories. Identifying characteristics have been changed to protect the privacy of those involved. Names that have been changed are indicated throughout the book by an asterisk (*).

Caveats

The information in this book is not intended to diagnose or treat any individual's health problems or conditions. Nor is it intended as medical or psychiatric advice, and it should not be construed as such. Please consult your own health care practitioner before beginning any unusual activity or discontinuing any aspect of treatment that you are currently undergoing.

None of the individuals or organizations involved with this book in any capacity holds out any promise of any therapeutic outcome for any individual through the Rubenfeld Synergy Method or any other healing art.

Glossary

The glossary and pronunciation guide, which begins on page 341, includes terms that may be unfamiliar to many readers as well as some that are used in a technical sense by Rubenfeld Synergists and other members of the healing professions.

First Impressions

OF RUBENFELD SYNERGY

THIRTY-FIVE YEARS AGO Ilana Rubenfeld was the sole practitioner of the body-oriented psychotherapy now known as the Rubenfeld Synergy Method. Anyone who experienced it did so at her hands. Since then Ilana has traveled around the country and the world, giving workshops that invariably include a demonstration session with one or more volunteer "clients." As these stories illustrate, observers of such demonstrations are often as deeply moved as the clients themselves.

Today many people get their first taste of Rubenfeld Synergy in the private office of a Certified Rubenfeld Synergist—one of over three hundred graduates of the professional training program that Ilana began in 1977. Most Synergists practice in the United States and Canada; a few in Mexico, Europe, and the Middle East.

During their training, students are required to practice Rubenfeld Synergy with many nonpaying clients under close supervision. The first story describes a session with one such client.

Synopses

The First Touch. At a workshop with Ilana, Millie learns to touch with "butterfly hands" and decides to apply for the training. Almost twenty years later she vividly remembers her first client's reaction to butterfly hands. This memory comes back to Millie as she touches each new client for the first time.

East Meets West: The Ninja–Rubenfeld Connection. Greg describes a weeklong workshop with Ilana. As her demonstration client, Greg makes contact with old, deeply buried anger. He discovers many similarities between Ilana and his martial arts teacher, the last grandmaster of Ninjutsu.

A Leap of Faith. In Suzanne's first session as a Rubenfeld Synergy client, she discovers feelings of guilt about her older brother's mental illness. She takes the first step in a long journey out of the depression that began in childhood.

Going Out on a Limb To Lighten Up. Estela describes her experience at a weekend Rubenfeld Synergy workshop. Later, in a private session, Estela faces some of her own painful memories. By working through the pain, she liberates the trapped energy in her body and begins to shed some emotional baggage.

Checking It Out. While researching a book about bodywork, Thomas has a session with Rob. During the session Thomas notices that his left and right sides feel different. This awareness leads to an exploration of his conflict between caution and desire to explore the world.

The First Touch

Millie Grenough

In 1978 I was working as an assistant to a clinical psychologist in New Haven, Connecticut, and was a trainee in a Gestalt theory and practice program. As part of the Gestalt training, we traveled to Greenwich Village in New York City to spend a morning with a woman named Ilana Rubenfeld. Our Gestalt trainers told us that Rubenfeld had devised a new method of therapy 'that paid attention to bodies as well as minds.

My introduction that morning to what is now known as the Rubenfeld Synergy Method intrigued me for personal and professional reasons. During the first thirty years of my very religious life, I had effectively ignored the realities of my body in favor of more "spiritual" matters. Then, after I left the church at the age of thirty, I spent ten years giving my body the chance to catch up on what it had never experienced. Often during these years it was more convenient to leave my mind elsewhere. Now approaching age forty I realized that my body, mind, and spirit were not very familiar with each other. I wanted to learn about myself and gain more insight into my profession, so I decided to apply for Ilana's next training class.

One of the requirements for acceptance into the training was attendance at a weekend workshop—to give us applicants a chance to "taste" the Rubenfeld Synergy Method and to give Ilana a chance to look us over. I signed up for a winter weekend at Wainwright House in Rye, New York, where I participated with about thirty other people in experiences that were—for me at the time—slightly bizarre.

I remember the first hands-on exercise. Ilana invited us to work with a partner to experiment with two different ways of touching. First we would put our hands on the shoulder of our partner with the intention of changing something about him—his posture or breathing or whatever. Then we would remove our hands, shake them out, and step away before approaching our partner with a different intention: simply being there with what Ilana called "listening hands." We would place our hands gently, but clearly, in contact with our partner's shoulder, without intending to change anything about him.

When my partner, Gabriel, put his hands on my shoulder with the intention of changing me, I remember stiffening against him. I felt handled and corrected—as if there were something wrong with my shoulders—and I didn't like it. Noticing my body's resistance, I decided to try another way and simply went limp, letting him do what he wanted. I didn't much like that either and was relieved when Gabriel stepped away at the end of the first part of the experiment. In the second part, when Gabriel touched me with the intention of listening with his hands, I noticed myself breathing with greater ease. I somehow felt seen by his hands and contacted in a way that invited my shoulder to breathe, to expand in any way it wanted to. Even though Gabriel was touching my shoulder, it didn't feel confined, and neither did I. In fact, I felt that his touch was giving me more room to be aware of my shoulder and myself.

Then we reversed roles so that I could be the toucher. When I touched Gabriel with the intention of changing him, I noticed that I focused on what was wrong with him and what my agenda was for fixing him. When I then approached him with listening hands, both my mind and my hands were more open. I felt curious about what I might find. I was open to surprises and to whatever information might be there.

In the ten minutes I spent doing this hands-on "first touch" experiment from both sides, I got the point. I was ready to begin the training.

In the first year of training, Ilana taught us many different ways of developing open, listening hands. In one vivid description she said, "Imagine a butterfly: how light it is, how delicate. Yet when this tiny butterfly touches down on one petal of a flower, the entire plant, even if it is six feet tall, vibrates."

We trainees practiced with each other for several months, always trying to clarify our intention and to come with open, curious hands. After several months we were ready to practice with "real people" outside of the training. Before our next training meeting we were to work with two or three people who knew nothing about Rubenfeld Synergy. Ilana gave us tips on working with these "practice clients." She advised us to use only very simple touching contacts and not attempt any emotional work. And to make it less likely that emotional material would emerge, she advised us not to work with friends, relatives, or emotionally unstable people.

On the train back to New Haven I was tired and excited. I thought about who I would ask to be my first practice client. Before I dozed off I thought, "Maybe Marie,* that friend of Barbara's. Yeah, Marie. I'll call her...."

Marie was small-boned, fragile-looking yet sturdy, about twenty-eight, with short, reddish blond hair and lively blue eyes. I felt safe practicing with Marie because she was a friend of two good friends of mine and seemed stable and self-assured. My friends told me that Marie loved dancing, was curious about new things, and would probably enjoy being a "practice client" for me.

I phoned Marie to see if she'd be interested. I explained to her that I was at the stage in my training where I could begin practicing with people outside the training program. I told her that I would simply be placing my hands on various parts of her body, that she would keep all her clothes on, and that, after the half-hour session, I would ask her for feedback. She thought it sounded interesting. We arranged to meet at our friend Barbara's house the next Wednesday evening.

During the next couple of days, I prepared myself by practicing my "listening hands" touch on myself, my cat, and various objects in my apartment. Wednesday finally arrived and I hustled home from work, showered, and changed into what I thought were appropriate Rubenfeld Synergy clothes: fresh, clean, comfortable cottons. Since I didn't yet have a padded, massage-type table, I rolled up an exercise mat and brought along a new sheet. At Barbara's suggestion I set up my mat in an out-of-the-way room. After taking a few minutes to collect myself, I went to invite Marie in.

Marie listened as I again explained what we would be doing. I told her that my intention was only to practice touch and not to explore any emotional material. I said that if anything happened that wasn't comfortable for her, or even if she felt that something might happen, to please let me know. I checked if she wanted to ask me anything before we began. She seemed bright-eyed and curious, but asked no questions.

She lay down on her back on the mat. I knelt near her head, warmed my hands, and began my first touch. Marie breathed calmly and seemed receptive. A minute passed. Then, to my great surprise, Marie began crying quietly, her tears running over her cheeks and wetting the new sheet.

My initial reaction was panic. I thought, "Oh my God, what have I done? Have I hurt her? Did I do something I shouldn't have done?" Then my training kicked in and reminded me to simply stay in contact with Marie without crowding her, to keep breathing and wait. I remembered that it was best to keep things simple. I let my hands stay in contact and didn't say anything.

Marie cried quietly for a minute or two. When I felt that it was okay to talk, I remembered a key, all-purpose question Ilana had suggested we use. I asked, very softly, "Marie, what are you experiencing now?"

She continued crying and explained tremblingly, "This is the first time anyone has ever touched me without wanting something back."

I have no clear memory of the rest of that first session. My only recollection is that Marie cried some more and that her body alternated between sobbing contractions and almost reluctant releases of tension. I noticed in her fragile features a look that was close to shell-shocked. At the end of the session I thanked Marie, asked for her feedback, and told her she could call me later if she wanted to ask any questions or check in with me. Then I asked Marie if there was anything she wanted to take with her from the evening. She said, "Yeah. I want to be more gentle with myself."

That was nineteen years ago. I don't know where Marie is now or if she remembers that first Rubenfeld Synergy touch. I know that I do.

Since then many a client has come into and out of my office. I can see some of their faces now: John, a fifty-nine-year-old businessman who was terrified of having another heart attack and had no idea of how to relax...thirty-five-year-old Linda, who'd had two husbands and many lovers but had never been held by her mother and was afraid of touch...twenty-eight-year-old Tom, who coped with his chronic physical pain and long-standing unhappiness by using a variety of drugs, perfecting his stand-up comedy routines, and attempting suicide from time to time...successful executive Louise, who at age forty was going through fertility treatments to try for a first pregnancy...college student Benita, who as a teenager had been abused and was now experiencing frequent nightmares and difficulties with her boyfriend...and vivacious Trudy, who, after nursing her husband through the final years of his long illness, began tap-dancing lessons on her sixtieth birthday and was herself diagnosed with cancer shortly afterward....

As I open my hands to make the first touch with each new client, Marie's words come back to me. "This is the first time anyone has ever touched me without wanting something back."

With this first touch—open, safe, and listening—the journey begins. There is time and room for anything. None of us knows where the journey will lead.

East Meets West:

THE NINJA–RUBENFELD CONNECTION

Greg Kowalski

I had mixed emotions the morning I first met Ilana. I was happy to be at Omega but annoyed that my girlfriend and I had apparently signed up for the wrong workshop! One of our friends had been urging us to do a "synergy" workshop, so when I saw the Rubenfeld Synergy workshop in the Omega catalog, we signed up. By the time we discovered that it was not the same synergy our friend was gung-ho about, it was too late to change our plans.

There was a lot more to my mixed emotions than just having signed up for the wrong kind of synergy. Life hadn't been going so well since my return from Japan, where I had spent four years training with Hatsumi-sensei, the last authentic grandmaster of the once secret Japanese Ninja [practitioners of an ancient martial art—*Ed.*]. Readjusting to life in the United States was a challenge.

I was battling chronic fatigue and other physical ailments, and there were some major problems in my relationship with Sharon, the woman with whom I was attending the workshop. I had recently left my stressful job—in the middle of a recession—to devote full time to my Ninjutsu school. All told, I was beginning to regret having left Japan.

The workshop started with Ilana, an animated, red-haired woman, warming the crowd up with some jokes. Then she had us work in pairs, doing basic sensitivity and energy games. Unfortunately I reacted so strongly against Sharon, my partner in this exercise, that I stopped playing. The exercise brought up every negative emotion I'd had toward her in the last six months, and then some. It turned into a pretty rough morning for both of us.

"Hava Nagila"

That afternoon, however, things started to change. Ilana set up a bodywork table in the center of our group and asked for a volunteer. A rather large gentleman came up and lay on the table. Ilana worked her way around his body, holding various parts gently, and began talking with him. Before long I was seeing him "regress" to his youth in Israel and reexperience some family difficulties that had taken place around the time of his bar mitzvah.

It was pretty impressive to watch. Perhaps fifty or more of us sat or stood, watching and empathizing with this man/boy on the table. It is hard to convey the energy in the room, the depth of our feelings as we observed this process. Many were holding back tears; others were wiping their eyes. The energy grew heavier as he relived his pain. I started to lose track of time.

Then Ilana shifted the conversation and began to help him to reconstruct and alter his experience of the past. With Ilana's gentle coaching and support, he began picking people out of the crowd to play the parts of different family members. I recall being impressed and surprised at his ability to be so present in the room, actively directing this scenario, yet still enough in the past to have it be real for him. Somewhere during this transition period, something else started to shift. Without ever denying what had happened or trivializing his pain, Ilana managed to help him get some different perspectives on the event that had affected him so profoundly through the years. She slipped a joke or two seamlessly into the dialogue between them, and he responded in kind. They continued setting the scene, preparing for a retake of his bar mitzvah. In the process it seemed to me that the heaviness and pain in the air had started to lessen, as if someone had opened a door or a window and a gentle breeze was blowing into the room.

The next thing I knew, the man was standing up on the table singing his bar mitzvah! As if a spell had been broken, the hall full of strangers soon began singing and laughing and dancing. Well, I wasn't dancing or singing, but I was looking around wide-eyed and shaking my head in mild amazement. I had been around a lot of weird parties in my day but this had to be one of the strangest! What had been such a painful, heavy session had erupted into a celebration of joy. Ilana turned from therapist to disc jockey, digging out every kind of music, from Yiddish to reggae, and the party continued until it was time for dinner. Unbelievable! As we walked up the stairs to the cafeteria, I got a good look at our volunteer and was struck by his appearance. His eyes sparkled and his face absolutely glowed. I began to think that maybe this week wouldn't be such a waste after all.

There was a lot of discussion that evening, people comparing notes, talking about how easily so many of us had been drawn into the man's session and had experienced so much emotion with a stranger. Jewish or not, male or female, we had all been touched by some part of it or another—what some might call universal themes of suffering, which know no nationality, race, religion, or gender and seem to come up in different fashions and flavors. The feelings of abandonment and rejection, whether real or only misperceived by a young person, had struck the chords of identity and empathy in all of us. Older men spoke of similar experiences with their bar mitzvahs, confirmations, or other significant milestones of adolescence. Others, women as well as men, told of how the session had recalled the experiences of their sons or nephews or had touched something in their own lives.

Waking the Dragon

The next morning, we sat or stood around the bodywork table, listening to Ilana talk. "So," she said as she began turning around, "would anyone like to volun…" She turned to find me standing directly in front of her. "But didn't you just have a session this morning?"

I had in fact taken the leap and had a session before breakfast with one of her staff people. "Yes, but I've got plenty."

"Ohhh. So you have plenty. All right!"

And so I came to be on my back, on the table, surrounded by people I didn't know. Except for Sharon. Her presence was, of course, a cause of concern for me as I imagined what might come up during the session. Still, there I was, briefing Ilana and the room on my "issues," telling her how I had been struggling with depression and unable to feel any other emotion for quite some time—as if everything were jammed up inside. Anger, it seemed, might be a major factor—anger unexpressed despite countless therapy sessions ranging from struggling to call up feelings of joy, to yelling, pillow-beating, and punching through stacks of pine boards. I had come to know a lot about myself and certainly a great deal about my childhood, my family issues, and all sorts of reasons and causes for my depression. Supposedly I knew enough to begin transforming all this understanding into different ways of being in my life. Yeah, I had all the tools for making changes. But nothing had changed. In fact, whatever "it" was, anger or whatever, it seemed to have a certain disdain for therapists and refused to be a party to anything as patronizing as pillow beating or other ragework. An artful dodger, it seemed to delight in toying with the so-called experts. I felt it watching and waiting, as was I, to see if this woman could do on me, too, what seemed to be some pretty powerful magic.

"What nice toes you have. Look at this one! What happened here?" She had discovered my big toe, bent and scarred from a few too many blocked kicks in my martial arts career.

"Rough life, I guess."

"Yes, I see that."

I was very aware of how tense I was becoming—surrounded by strangers, with Sharon watching and both of us nervous about what might come out. I felt that my life, my psychological life at least, was riding on this session. After so many years of disappointments and frustrations, was this something that might actually work? Or would it be just another tease, another carrot on a stick to keep the jackass moving? A lot was going on for me as Ilana stayed with my feet, playing with my toes.

"Such nice little piggies. Do you remember how that goes? 'This little piggy...'? What did this little piggy do?"

You've got to be kidding! I felt myself cringing. I may have groaned audibly. "Cutesy" is one thing I do not do. Yet I had asked to be on the table, so eventually, with a great deal of resistance, I started to play.

"Market."

"Right. Now say the whole thing. 'This little...'"

I made a face and eventually squeezed out the phrase, "This

little piggy went to market."

It was tough. The room was getting tense, warm, and more than a little uncomfortable as she teased me on to the next toe. And the next. And the next until we finished. A sigh of relief.

Oh no! She started over again on the other foot. I gave a big sigh and felt my shoulders drop to the table as I resigned myself to my fate with a silent, "God, I feel stupid!" After the second foot was finished, she started all over again on the first. This time we had to change things a little, making sure each little piggy got something nice.

"This one stayed home. And what did he do while he stayed home?" she went on in a singsong tone as if I were a little child. Arrrgh!

"Did he do something fun? The other one had roast beef. What could this one have?"

Oh, come on, lady, give me a break! I felt my stomach flutter. My abdominal muscles started to spasm and I realized something inside was starting to stir. It felt uncomfortable…and familiar. Oh yes, I recognized it all right. It had come up a time or two in the past in *inpi* [sweat lodge] ceremonies. The first time had been in a lodge with Wallace Black Elk. Like some powerful spiritual expectorant, the sweat had broken something loose—something not very nice—and as it came to the surface I had been able to sense it, feel it, and do battle with it, so to speak. What a very long, exhausting night that had been, and here "it" was again, squirming inside at having to play this stupid little game! I felt another spasm through my stomach and realized I'd been had. I lifted my head and gave Ilana a look, part hatred, part amusement, and shook my head in grudging respect.

"You're good, lady," I said quietly. And we continued with the little piggies as I became more and more aware of something powerful stirring and squirming inside.

I began to lose track, fading in and out as she got me talking of my childhood, getting me to remember, to imagine what certain things had been like. I felt myself slipping into an altered state, my voice changing. I was acutely aware of some struggle taking place inside me. I was resenting Ilana, her questions, even the tone of her voice. Caught between embarrassment at being made to play these silly games and the desire to see this through, I realized my focus had been drifting. And all the while, part of my attention was on whatever it was that was moving inside, as if it were being poked and prodded, becoming more and more uncomfortable and annoyed, until it began looking around for the source—like a sleeping dog, teased and baited until it could no longer ignore its tormentor. Perhaps a dragon would be a more appropriate metaphor, a leviathan stirring in the mud and muck of my psyche.

Our conversation was taking me back in time to some unpleasant situations that I knew all too well. God knows they had been talked about often enough. They must have been resolved and released by now. Yet my responses came slowly, after long, tense silences. My voice was quiet and angry. I seemed to be enveloped in darkness. Inside was dark as well, and eventually I realized that whatever it was that was stirred up inside was now on its way to the surface.

In an instant I was aware of many things on many levels. It was anger, or at least it came with anger. Rage was more like it. And what was more shocking was the feeling that what I was aware of was just the point man, the vanguard of something greater, something much more primal welling up from beneath it. It felt in fact as if something were rumbling from below me, from inside the bowels of the Earth itself. I was jolted with the awareness that I was sitting on a volcano of dark, violent energy that was about to explode!

There was no way I would be able to control this. It was nothing to be channeled, "dialogued" with, or tamed. I knew that when it reached the surface I would be gone, out of control, and I was flooded with images of the aftermath: the massage table in pieces, Ilana lying like a broken doll, windows shattered and the people in the room broken and injured, as if by a bomb blast, and flashing lights, sirens, and ambulances in the wake of the eruption. I knew there was no way I could let go. I would be overwhelmed, swallowed up in something that felt almost evil—a blind rage exploding through twenty years of hard-core martial arts training. This was not safe. I began searching for the brakes. I brought all my will to bear, resisting against the upward rush. Finally it slowed, eventually halting, the dragon face snarling up from below before turning back to sink once more into the darkness.

Ilana was waiting for me to answer. What had she been saying? How long ago was it? The singsong quality of her voice had changed at some point. The cute games had been dropped and we were speaking very slowly and softly of events from my childhood.

With difficulty I, too, became a partner in directing a rescripting process. When it was over this time, however, there was no dancing and no singing. As I stepped off the table, I felt as if I were in shock. When I began to look around, I saw everyone in the room transfixed—some in tears—all quite obviously affected by whatever had been going on during my session. A member of her staff had participated in this rescripting and Ilana had me go outside with him and another man to walk around and feel the Earth under my feet. I felt at the same time like a young boy and like someone very ancient. Walking was like a new experience. I felt the ground as if for the first time. I felt exhausted as well, light and heavy at the same time, totally spent.

Throughout the day members of the group approached me to share their experiences of watching my session. *Watching* is perhaps not an accurate term for it. More often than not it seemed as if somehow everyone participated in every session throughout the week—and was touched and affected as well, judging from the feedback I received.

One older gentleman came to thank me and told me his story: He had arrived at registration that day only to find that the workshop he had come for had been canceled. He had not been notified and he was infuriated. Having taken the time off and come all this way, he grudgingly chose Ilana's workshop as a substitute, even though it was already in its second day. Unhappy and unaware, he had walked into the middle of my session. He shared with me how hearing and watching my session had brought up a lot of emotion and insight about his relationship with his son; it had touched him very deeply.

As it turned out he and I each had a remarkable time that week, even though we both had come to the wrong workshop. I certainly got in touch with the emotions that had evaded all prior approaches. My only regret is that I had a session with Ilana so early in the week. By the end of the workshop, having watched her more, I would have trusted her to handle what I had perceived to be the imminent explosion of rage. Even though I had shut down that part of the process, the session had much more impact—and seemed to be much more real to me—than any previous therapeutic experience.

The Rubenfeld–Ninja Connection

As I went through the rest of the week, integrating my own experience and watching new demonstration sessions every day, each very different from the others, I was repeatedly amazed. I kept saying to Sharon, "I'm looking at a five-foot-tall, red-haired, Jewish-grandmother version of Hatsumi-sensei." I could clearly see that what Ilana was doing in her work was remarkably similar to what I had learned—in a different manifestation, of course—in my training with the Ninja.

Just as a Ninja rides the attacker's energy and movement rather than "doing" a technique on or to him, Ilana follows the client's flow instead of directing or instructing him. The grandmaster offered the means to a greater level of awareness—a fundamental requirement for creating change in our lives. He led people to the doors and mirrors that could serve them in their personal growth. It is of course up to the individual to choose to look in the mirrors or go through the doors—or, I now realized, to explore the alternatives offered so subtly in Ilana's open-ended approach.

As I watched Ilana work I could hear Hatsumi-sensei say in his accented English, "Don't grab. Don't grab. Light touch, light touch. Don't try. Don't think. Let it happen." I saw in both masters the transcendence of the rigid pursuit of dogma in favor of being in the "spirit" of the moment—the proverbial "be here now," manifesting continually through the ever-changing interactions of the people involved in "the Dance."

I came away from that week telling my friends it was the only thing in the last twenty years that had impressed me as profoundly as my initial encounters with the Ninja grandmaster.

Epilogue

I still felt that way half a year later, when I arrived at Ilana's brownstone in Greenwich Village to begin learning her art. It has now been four years since that week at Omega, and in another month I will join the small group of people who have been trained and certified by Ilana to do this work.

Over the past few years of training I have remained amazed at the depth of our work and the powerful, positive impact it has had with my many practice clients. I realize, too, that like the Ninja's art Rubenfeld Synergy is at once refreshingly open and deeply grounded, a process of never-ending learning and growth that will always lead to more. I have continued to be impressed by Ilana and her abilities, yet even more so by her making this process available for others to learn. Significantly, it is the process itself that becomes the ultimate teacher.

I had been wanting for quite some time to train in a healing art—to complement my training in the martial arts and provide the kind of balance that would have been part of Ninjutsu training in ages past. I had been exploring different healing modalities, but until that week at Omega I had yet to experience anything that inspired my inner vision to say, "This is it." Discouraged in my search, for the moment I had given up looking.

And then a series of events, "errors," and coincidences led me to sign up for the wrong workshop, to find myself lying on a table in a room full of strangers, reciting a nursery rhyme. . . .

A Leap of Faith

Suzanne Gluck-Sosis

It's 1979, four years after the death of my husband of nearly twenty years, and I'm still seeking ways to become a more whole person. I've been in talk therapy intermittently for over twenty-five years, since before I met my husband. Although my levels of self-doubt, anxiety, and self-hatred have lessened considerably, I still have a deep-down judgment about myself as "bad."

Attending a conference of the Association of Humanistic Psychology, I see that Ilana Rubenfeld is giving a workshop on the Rubenfeld Synergy Method. It sounds intriguing and I ask myself, "Shall I chance it?" A part of me hesitates: "What will I discover?" I am fearful of coming face to face with something I might not want to know. Another part of me says, "Go for it! Take a risk! What have you got to lose? You're miserable—lonely and confused, empty," although only my therapist knows I have such feelings. I sign up for the workshop.

After an introduction, Ilana asks for a volunteer client from the audience. A woman jumps up, goes to the front, and gets on the table. I breathe a sigh of relief and regret. (After eighteen years I've forgotten the details of the demonstration, but I remember my astonishment at what I saw: the compassion, validation, and empathy; the laughter and tears; and the resolution of a troubling issue in the woman's life—all in forty-five minutes.)

At lunchtime I think, "I must experience this method. Maybe it will make a difference in how I feel." I take a leap of faith and seek out one of Ilana's graduates. Don* agrees to give me a session and asks if I have any questions. I am eager and hopeful but I have no questions yet. "I just want to experience being on the table." So Don invites me to lie on my back on the table in an empty workshop room. "Allow yourself to take a few deep breaths in and out. Scan your body to see where there might be some tension. If there is, just notice it; don't try to fix it." I breathe deeply, wondering what's to come, hoping I'll do "the right thing" and not make a fool of myself. Don's voice is soothing, soft, neutral with a hint of a twinkle. I feel my body softening.

"Is there something you need to tell me?"

My throat tightens a bit—I find myself telling him about my family of origin. Tears flow freely down my face as I choke out, "I feel angry, hurt, ashamed, and constantly guilty. I'm remembering my family when I was a kid. I hate them! My brother is manic-depressive; my parents are depressed—full of uncertainty and doubt, not knowing what to do. Somehow I feel I'm to blame for everything."

Don makes a sympathetic sound. "Tell me more about how you feel."

"I am furious with everyone! No one knows how to help my

brother, Roy. He is misunderstood—my parents and other relatives are afraid of him and try to control him. Roy is unmanageable. He is finally diagnosed as manic-depressive, and is hospitalized, at age sixteen. I feel ashamed and guilty somehow—it's my fault: I cannot save him."

"How old are you when he is hospitalized?"

"I am eight years old."

"If you are eight and he sixteen when he is first hospitalized, then Roy is eight years old when you are born. You are an infant, you are a child, powerless to do anything to help your brother. How can you be responsible for his illness?"

I am silent as this idea slowly sinks in.

After a pause Don asks, "Would you agree to do an experiment?"

"What do you have in mind?"

"Tell Roy how you feel about him."

I start tentatively. "I love you, Roy." It takes a while for me to get the hang of it. "You are the live one in this family. You taught me to love music, literature, art, social issues. I think Mom and Dad and our aunts and uncles are not helping you. They are making you worse. They don't understand you. I can take care of you better. But I'm too little. I'm only two and you are ten."

As I talk Don places his hands under my left hip and requests that I focus on it. He moves to my right hip, my legs, allowing the body to release the energy in each area. I can sense a shift in bodily sensations. There is less heaviness in my head; it feels lighter, airier. I don't sound so bad. A flood of relief passes through me. "Maybe I'm not as horrid as I feel."

Don asks me what I remember about Roy. "Oh, he is so good-looking—blond hair, blue eyes, long lashes—and so charming. He is full of ideas when he is not being manic or depressive. He sings Gilbert and Sullivan—he is Frederic in *Pirates of Penzance,* and I sing Mabel when he practices at home. I love it! It fills me with warmth, light, and joy to be sharing this rehearsal with him."

Don continues to gently touch, hold, and move my arms, legs, back, hips, head, and neck. I feel more and more relaxed, sinking into the table. Feeling open, clear, and free, I smile and laugh. Don has an ironic sense of humor, which appeals to me. He says, "You move gracefully on the table."

I giggle. "I am a dancer…in my soul."

Don seems to understand and empathize with what I'm saying. I feel safe with him—able to tell him almost anything without fear of being criticized or punished. So when he suggests I dance, I am happy to get off the table and do so. I dance without self-consciousness. I twirl, spin, leap, run, turn, filled with excitement and light. I dare not look at him while I dance for fear I will see disapproval in his eyes. I finish and then turn to gaze directly at him. His eyes are shining with appreciation. "That is wonderful," he says, smiling.

I am overjoyed. I feel aglow with love and warmth. Silently I vow to apply to the training program.

What did not come out in that first session with Don—and what I was unable to express openly for many years afterward— was my terror that I, too, might be crazy. Gradually, over several years of personal and group Rubenfeld sessions and supervision, I came to see how my depression had been keeping me at a safe distance from this fear, and I became more comfortable with myself. By the time I met my second husband a few years ago, I was finally ready to risk a new relationship. With the help of his unconditional acceptance and unerring love, I have found the courage to face my lifelong fear and have freed myself from its grip.

Going Out on a Limb To Lighten Up

Estela M. Hernandez

I first met Ilana Rubenfeld in the spring of 1993. Around that time I had changed careers, from a nursing practitioner in clinical research to a college educator in the health-allied sciences. Because of my interest in holistic health care, I picked up a bulletin from the New York Open Center one day and came across an article on a workshop Ilana was about to present: "Out on a Limbic.[1]" I was immediately intrigued by the title, which I understood to mean being out on a limb with your emotions. I had spent many hours with critically and terminally ill patients, and knew what it felt like to be "out on a limbic." The title spoke directly to my heart and piqued my curiosity about what Ilana

---

[1] The limbic system is a set of deep cortical structures in the brain, associated with emotion, memory, affect, and motivation.

might have to say about healing. So I enrolled in her weekend workshop, not having a clue that what I was about to experience would profoundly change the direction of my life.

In the first demonstration that Ilana gave of the Rubenfeld Synergy Method, she had a group of about thirty attendees form a circle around a padded table. She explained that she wanted to work with someone willing to explore the deeper issues surrounding physical and/or emotional discomfort, rather than with someone who just wanted her to "fix" the pain. Al,* who was a bear of a man, volunteered to lie down on the table, while the rest of us settled down in our seats to watch and listen.

In a soft voice, Ilana asked Al questions as she gently touched his hips and shoulders in turn. Within a few minutes I saw each leg and shoulder drop, relaxing deeper into the padding. Then Al closed his eyes and began to tell his story. On that day, in a room full of strangers, he revealed the pain and horror of his childhood. He became the little boy who had witnessed his father drinking and beating his mother and had experienced verbal and physical abuse from his mother. To survive he had told himself over and over again, "I'm big and tough. I can take it." This outwardly powerful man was speaking from the place of a lonely, scared, and defenseless child.

The session lasted an hour and fifteen minutes. During that time I was acutely aware of an increase in the room temperature and a sense of timelessness. I observed the revealing tear-stained faces of the group; I, too, was deeply moved and felt the depth of my own childhood pain. As a health professional, I had often contributed to team discussions of the psychotherapeutic treatment plan for a patient, but never had I witnessed a session anything like this—without an authority figure dictating what the client must do to get better. What I saw was a skilled and compassionate woman guiding and empowering this man to listen to the wisdom of his body. As I listened I felt a crushing heaviness in my own chest, and it shocked me into realizing how much healing I needed in my own life. I had never been tempted in the past to undergo therapy for myself. But after this session I was absolutely convinced that I had to be part of this program, which empowered people to explore their internal healing abilities rather than look to "outside experts" to do it for them.

When the workshop came to a close, I stayed behind to ask Ilana how I could learn to do the Rubenfeld Synergy Method. As she suggested, I applied for admission into the training program beginning that fall. Upon acceptance I began once-a-week private sessions with a Rubenfeld Synergist in order to start my own self-exploration. As eager as I was to learn this hands-on healing method, I was not looking forward to digging into the depths of my own emotional baggage! I knew I would have to summon the courage to face my own fears, while continuing to work and function in my everyday life. It was in this frame of mind that I entered my first session with Marilyn*—feeling anxious, cautious, curious, and maybe even a little courageous.

Marilyn's office was small, with a teal-colored padded table on one side and a small wooden table and two chairs on the other. She and I spoke for a few minutes, and I told her a little bit about my professional background. Then I shared with her that I had pain throughout my body, particularly in my legs and ankles, due to rheumatoid arthritis. When she asked if I would like to go to the table, I consented. Initially I had been surprised by how young she looked, but by this time I was feeling more comfortable with her, and I liked her upbeat spirit.

Once I was on the table, Marilyn instructed me to softly close my eyes and bring my awareness to my body. As I did so I noticed the tension in my muscles, my uncomfortable shortness of breath, and the anxious, rapid beating of my heart. I remember that Marilyn placed her hands around my left hip and instructed me to focus on that area, to notice what came up for me. I didn't know exactly what I was supposed to do, so I just tried to bring my attention to my hip. At first that was difficult, but then I started to imagine the placement of my bones. I began to see the shape of my pelvis, hip socket, and femur, and I noticed stiffness throughout my entire leg.

When Marilyn asked what I was experiencing, I told her what I'd noticed. Then she gently slid her hands down my entire leg and something startling happened. I didn't know what or how, but I felt my leg change and become loose and longer. She asked me what I noticed about my left leg and how it compared to the right one. My right leg felt stiff and contracted, smaller and shorter than the left.

After I shared all this with Marilyn, she placed her hands around my right hip and instructed me to bring my awareness there. I remember thinking, "Thank God! I can do this. It's not so hard." Then all of a sudden, my mind went into a very dark place, into a void of darkness filled with hopelessness, despair, pain, and sorrow. I felt as if in a prison with no way out. I saw flashes of experiences I'd had as a teenager. I remember Marilyn's voice giving me support and encouraging me to stay in this fearful place a little longer. I was filled with tears and sorrow and shame. And I was deathly afraid.

In less than an hour's time I relived the helplessness of a lost love, the anguish, guilt, and shame of an abortion, the hopelessness of an attempted suicide, and the lonely despair of an abandoned teenage girl. I perceived these memories as black areas stuck in my pelvis, especially on the right side. I don't know how or where I found the strength to survive this painful experience, but I remember Marilyn as being with me all the way. I cried and cried and, perhaps for the first time, truly felt my broken heart.

At the end of the session I felt stunned and a little embarrassed. I needed a couple of minutes to compose myself before I could look at Marilyn. When I finally looked into her eyes, I saw no judgment or criticism, only compassion and understanding. I felt very grateful for her support and thanked her for helping me get through such a difficult journey. As I got off the table, I noticed my legs felt lighter and less painful. I also had a sense of calmness, and somehow my body felt very different.

Once I arrived home I tried to remember all that had occurred and to figure out exactly how I'd been able to go so deeply into myself. I finally had to give it up because my brain couldn't understand it. What I did realize is that I had gone through an experience like no other, and it was not because Marilyn had hypnotized me or forced me to imagine horrible things. Intuitively I knew I had felt and relived pain I hadn't been strong enough to experience before. Somehow I had retained all that emotional pain in my body, and until that day I was unaware of the magnitude of emotions that I was holding on to. That session marked the beginning of a deeper level of healing through increased awareness, a healing that continues to affect all aspects of my life.

Today, five years later, I continue my journey of self-exploration through Rubenfeld Synergy and share my knowledge and insights with my students, Synergy clients, colleagues, friends, and family. I've learned to forgive and love myself, as well as others, and to allow joy to enter my life. I have lightened up my former areas of darkness. And in allowing my light to shine through, I have become a model for others to do the same.

Today, when my friends hug me, they comment on how light my body feels. I laugh, knowing it's because I have dropped some heavy baggage from my life!

Checking It Out

Thomas Claire

*Thomas Claire, a practicing massage
therapist, had this session while
doing research for his book,* Bodywork.[1]

On a sunny April afternoon, I arrive at the apartment of Rob
Bauer, a practitioner and senior instructor of Rubenfeld Synergy.
Rob greets me at the door and shows me in. Inviting me to sit
opposite him, he takes a few minutes to get to know me. He asks
me what issues are going on for me right now. Which ones are
most important? What can he do to help me?

I explain that I'm in a period of great transition. I'm completing a number of projects that have been consuming my time for
the last several years. I feel a great sense of relief at this, for I've
been aware of the pressure, deadlines, and other stresses involved
in completing these projects. I also feel a great sense of freedom.

---

[1] Adapted from the chapter, "Rubenfeld Synergy Method: Touch Therapy Meets Talk
Therapy." By permission of William Morrow & Company, Inc., and Thomas Claire.

I've been feeling tied down. A major segment of my life is coming to completion; I'll be free to entertain other projects. I'm also thinking about moving, leaving the apartment in which I've been living and using my newfound freedom to drift for a while and take stock of my life. I'd like to travel the globe—Paris, India, Nepal, Central America. The idea, while exciting, is also stressful. I've lived in my present apartment for seven years. I feel secure and grounded there.

Rob explains that what I've shared gives us plenty of material with which to begin our hands-on work. He explains that I'll be lying down on a padded massage table in the middle of the room. I will remain clothed during the session. I've dressed in a T-shirt, sweatshirt, and loose-fitting sweat pants to be comfortable during the session. Rob asks me to remove my watch and anything I may have in the pockets of my pants.

I lie down on my back on the table and close my eyes while Rob stands at the head of the table. He asks me whether I prefer to be called Tom or Thomas. This seemingly simple question immediately unearths a conflict: I go by both Tom and Thomas. Family members and old friends call me Tom. I now prefer to be called Thomas, which is the name I use professionally. In response to Rob's query, I reply "Thomas."

Rob asks me to begin the session by becoming aware of my body and any sensations I may be experiencing. He asks me how my body feels as it meets the table. How does my head feel? Does it have a tendency to fall to one side? Is it as relaxed as it can be? What about my shoulders, my back, my arms? As he asks how my arms feel, I experience a tightness around my eyes. I wonder if he senses this when he asks his next question: "How does your face feel? Notice your breathing—not to change it, but just how it feels. Is it deep, full? How do your hips feel? Your legs? Your feet?"

He asks me to become aware of all these sensations without judging or trying to change anything.

Rob's voice is hypnotic. As he talks he seems to be both lulling me into relaxation and heightening my awareness. I am silent as I internally scan my body and feelings.

"I'm going to begin by gently touching your head," Rob says. He cradles the back of my head in his hands, just holding. "I'm just greeting you," he says. "I'm saying hello to you, and you're saying hello to me. We're getting to know one another on the level of touch. When you first came in, we got to know one another through talk. Now we're meeting through touch."

Rob lightly cradles my head for a short time, then he gently rolls it from side to side. He asks me to share with him what I'm feeling.

I explain that when I turn my awareness toward my body, I become conscious that the left side of my body seems to sink more deeply into the table. It feels more relaxed and open. I tell Rob that I get a feeling of support from the way he cradles my head, that his simple gesture of intentional, caring touch, just holding and listening, without doing anything, makes me feel that everything is all right. I say that I realize, from feeling supported in this way, how much I worry, am fearful and anxious about doing things right and being perfect, but now I feel that everything is okay. It is okay for me just to be here, now, as I am.

"Just to be here now, as you are; it's okay just to be here, now, as you are," Rob repeats. "Did you feel anything else that you want to share?"

I explain that I felt a stiffness in my neck—that as he rolled my head from side to side, it didn't seem to roll easily; it felt stiff and tight, not elastic.

Rob asks, "Is it fair to say that one side of your body feels more open and free, the other more cautious and guarded? And if so, does that mean anything to you?"

What Rob says seems to fit. It is obvious to me that my body is saying that one side is more open, the other more cautious. And when I think about my life situation, I feel it's true there, too. One part of me wants to be free, open, like a child playing outdoors on this idyllic spring day. Another side of me says, no, you can't do that; you have to stay inside and work. You can't be free. Part of me wants to uproot myself and travel the globe; another part says, no, you have to stay put, you need security, you can't move.

Rob advances to the foot of the table. He gently rolls each of my legs. He asks me how they feel. I note that they feel heavy and leaden, like pieces of deadwood. I feel the same difference between right and left sides here as I did earlier: The right leg feels deader than the left.

"So the legs are telling us the same thing—one side is more open than the other," Rob says. He moves to the left side of the table. "Before we go any further, I'd like to make a contract with you. If anything feels at all uncomfortable to you, you're to let me know. Is that okay?"

The contract seems simple and more than fair to me. Rob continues, "I'm going to begin to work with your left side. Since that side is more open, it'll be easier to start there. I'm going to make a hip sandwich," he says, and I grin. "I'm going to put my hands on either side of your left hip." Rob places his left hand on top of my hip, his right under it. He holds for what seems like several minutes, then asks me to verbalize my feelings about what's happening. "You might experience these feelings as images, colors, or physical sensations. Whatever comes to you is okay."

"I'm feeling heat," I report. "When you first put your hands on my hip, I felt tremendous heat coming from your hands. But I also feel heat between them, in my own tissue. I'm feeling as though the tissue is expanding, that a tightness that was held there is releasing. It feels fuller, denser. I also feel my breath becoming much deeper. Almost as soon as you put your hands on my hip, my abdomen swelled up with deeper breath. Especially the lower abdomen, below the navel in the pelvic basin. It felt like a big football swelling up."

Rob says, "You felt the heat of my hands and you felt the warmth of your own tissue. It felt denser to you." He releases his hands and jostles my hip a little as it softens. He takes his hands and passes them down my left leg in a broad, sweeping, whooshing motion. When he gets to my feet, he jostles my left leg gently back and forth and asks me how it feels. I tell him it feels as free and loose as a chicken leg that's cooked until you can rotate the bone easily.

Rob moves to my right side and makes a hip sandwich around my right hip. He asks me to share what I'm feeling there. Again, I feel the heat of his hands and the area filling up. But what I'm most aware of is how empty this area feels. Even with the heat and sense of growing fullness it seems caved in, hollowed out, in relation to my left hip. My right leg has a tendency to turn out, and I can feel how flat this makes the area around the hip feel, almost flat like a piece of plywood, as opposed to the roundness and fullness on my left side.

"Where do you feel this flatness?" Rob asks me. "Just in the hip, or in other parts of your body?"

"All the way down to my knee," I answer, "and up through my waist area to my right shoulder, too."

Rob releases my right hip, whooshing down to my foot again. He jostles my right leg from the foot, then my left leg. He asks me what I'm feeling.

The legs feel very different. They feel alive, vibrating, pulsating with energy. The right side still feels more restricted than the left, but both legs feel much more open than they did at the beginning of the session.

"So compared to each other, one side still feels more open, one side more cautious," Rob summarizes. "If you had to say which one felt more open, more willing to explore, travel, or let go, and which one felt more guarded, wanting safety, which would they be?"

"My left side is the more open and free; the right feels more tied down."

"That's the second time you've used the phrase 'tied down,'" Rob says. "It must mean something to you. If you were to say something to your hip, which one would you want to talk to and what would you ask?"

I ponder for a moment. "I'd talk to my right hip. I'd ask it why it felt tied down. Why it feels tight and restricted."

"Then why don't you try asking it," Rob urges. "The body is wise. Maybe it has an answer for you. Ask it: 'Hip, why do you feel tied down? Why are you tight and restricted?'"

"Why do you feel tied down, right hip?" I ask. "Why are you tight and restricted?" I feel a little self-conscious talking to my body in this way. At the same time, I'm beginning to feel a closer connection to my body. I feel as though it's offering answers at the same time I'm asking it questions.

"It tells me it's feeling left out, ignored," I explain to Rob. "It's always wanted to be free, to run and play."

Rob says, "If you're willing, perhaps you could ask it more questions, request more information."

All the while he's talking to me, Rob is moving his hands slowly, purposefully, gently. His tone of voice and quality of touch convey both concern and gentle, caring support. Now his hands are under my back, noodling in gentle pressing motions the muscles that run alongside my spine. At times he seems to be just listening and patiently waiting. As he reaches the area under my right shoulder blade, I'm aware of the tension and pain in my muscles. This is the area where I tend to hold my habitual tension, the place where I feel my aches and pains. Rob's touch is firm. It doesn't hurt physically, but I'm aware of a pain and sensitivity in the tissue. It feels like a burning sensation. I can't tell whether this pain is new, brought on by this session, or whether I'm just becoming aware of a pain that's always been there. I share these impressions with Rob.

He says, "Often, people become aware of pain during their sessions. Many people expect to feel relaxed and good. But I explain to them that this work often brings up pain. It's more like psychotherapy, making us aware of ourselves, than massage."

I listen to my body, to the pain and restriction I feel. I ask my right side why it feels tied down, restricted, ignored. It tells me that this feeling goes back a long way, to my childhood, to the days when feelings didn't yet have the words to express themselves. It's connected to my feeling that I couldn't just be me. My parents' love always seemed qualified, as though they were telling me, "You can be anybody you want to be so long as it's what we want you to be."

"So your right hip got tied down," Rob says. "Because you couldn't be who you wanted to be, it got tied down."

Rob asks me to roll over onto my right side. He's manipulating my right torso and shoulder area from underneath my body in this side-lying position.

"What would you like to say to your right side?" Rob asks.

"I'd like to tell it that it's okay to be just who it is, without any limitation or precondition."

"Then try it," Rob suggests. "Try saying it to your right side."

I say to my right side, "It's okay to be who you are, just as you are. I'll love you anyway."

"How does that feel?" Rob asks.

My right side doesn't believe it. I've said the words, but I don't feel it in my body. It still feels tight. My body doesn't buy it.

"Maybe this part of your body doesn't trust what you say," Rob says. "Maybe it's been lied to before. Maybe your parents told it they loved it just as it was, but then didn't let it be who it was."

What Rob, or my body, is saying to me is very powerful. I realize all the mixed messages I've gotten, how many conflicting memories and feelings about myself are recorded in my body's tissues. I've been through many years of talk psychotherapy with several talented practitioners. I know many things at the intellectual level. But now I'm *feeling* them in the tissues of my body, and they don't lie. They won't accept something they don't believe.

Rob is working with my right shoulder. He stretches my arm in a circular rotating motion. I'm aware of how tight it feels, how my arm doesn't really want to go above my collarbone.

"What do you feel here in your right shoulder?" Rob asks. "What's going on for you?"

I tell him how tight this shoulder feels. "Yes," he agrees. "Why don't you try asking your shoulder what's going on, what it's feeling, why it's so tight?"

I ask my shoulder and it replies, "I can't even give you an answer because I've never been allowed to think for myself. I'm tight because I haven't been given the freedom to think."

"Your shoulder can't even think, and you want to make it go around the world with you?" Rob jokes. "No wonder it's confused. Why don't you ask it how it feels about that?"

I ask my shoulder, and it replies, "That's absurd. It's absurd that a grown man feels he can't think for himself and that he's going off around the world anyway. It's absurd, but true."

As I talk Rob continues to employ gentle jostling, stretching, twisting motions. I'm aware of a pain, a tight painful tissue, that stretches from my right hip all the way to my shoulder blade. It crosses the area where I feel the habitual pain in my right mid-back. It seems somehow connected to this pain I'm feeling. Rob reinforces my awareness that the pain I feel is not only in the hip; it is also connected to a larger pattern of holding throughout my body. He asks me to roll over onto my left side.

"What would you like to say to your right shoulder?" he asks, as he resumes the gentle stretching and jostling of my right side and shoulder. "Maybe this holding is related to a child inside of Thomas, to the child Thomas," Rob suggests. "Is there anything the adult Thomas would like to say to the child Thomas?"

I answer, "The adult Thomas wants to tell the child, 'Thomas, it's okay for you not to think. It's okay for you just to be.' Not to know what's going to happen next. To accept the fact that it's okay not to be perfect. That there's no one right way of doing anything. To trust to the universe."

"Maybe the child Thomas is afraid," Rob suggests, "afraid that the adult Thomas is going to give up all his security and run off around the world. But maybe the child Thomas doesn't understand that the adult Thomas is responsible, that he's not going to take any risks that would hurt the child Thomas. That it's possible to be free and open, responsibly, without being hurt."

As Rob offers these suggestions, I can feel and see the child Thomas. Somewhere in the tissue of my body I see a small but bright white light, the child Thomas, who is afraid. I realize this is a part of myself I've ignored all these years. What is so powerful about connecting with this part of myself is the immediacy of the feeling. In the tissue beneath Rob's hands, I can feel the child within. I realize I have an opportunity to establish a partnership with my child self—the adult Thomas and the child Thomas can support one another and travel together in security, not in fear.

Rob concludes work on my shoulder by stretching the area between it and the pectoral muscles of the chest. Then he asks me to roll onto my back again. He moves to the foot of the table and jostles my legs. Now they feel really free, open, and full. He lifts my legs to position them at a forty-five-degree angle to my body, so that my lower back is supported. He places one hand on my lower stomach and the other on my breastbone in what seems like a final balancing act. He asks me to open my eyes when I'm ready and to share any feelings with him.

As I open my eyes I notice the pale rose color of the paint on his ceiling. It mirrors the sense of peace and calm I feel. I tell Rob how much more relaxed I feel, especially my neck. How my lower back makes deeper and more secure contact with the table. How appreciative I feel to have met the child Thomas and gotten to know him better.

Rob asks me to gently roll over onto whatever side beckons me as I rise to a seated position. I move onto my right side, the poor, ignored child side, much more in tune with it. Rob suggests that I sit quietly for a moment to let myself readjust to being upright. He then asks me to walk around the room to see how I feel.

What I'm most aware of is how much I feel my lower body. My awareness after bodywork is often in the upper part of my body. Now I now feel very grounded; my buttocks and legs feel heavy; my feet deeply rooted in the Earth. I share this with Rob and tell him I feel this is just the beginning of a process, that there is still much work to be done.

"Of course it's just the beginning," Rob agrees. "I work with some clients for weeks or months and others for years. Often as we work, issues emerge that are different from the ones that brought the client to see me in the first place, and we work on the new ones."

Rob reassures me that the issues raised during our session are not unique to me. My feelings, such as that of not being loved for who I really am, reflect universal human concerns. I feel further healing through my connection to the greater pool of humanity.

In parting, Rob says, "I hope your work pressures aren't so great that you can't allow yourself to process what we've done, and find some time for personal enjoyment today. Remember the part of yourself that wants to do that."

When I leave Rob's apartment, I notice that the day is still warm and brilliantly sunny. This is the first warm day after one of the longest and coldest winters in decades. I allow myself the spontaneous freedom to enjoy a stroll in the sun, secure in the knowledge that I will be responsible enough to make the time later to accomplish whatever work goals I might have.

I feel much freer. I feel that it's okay to be just me and not worry that I should be perfect. Later that day, this sense of openness is reflected in my work as a professional massage therapist. As I give a massage to a regular weekly client I feel more free to improvise, not following a preset treatment plan but moving with the flow of the moment. My client notices it, too: "Is it the day or is it you?" he asks. "I'm absolutely melting into the table. This is one of your best massages—you'll have to record it and duplicate it again."

That evening I dream about moving. I dream I've rented out part of my house to another man, a brother or a twin. I'm ready to move, but he isn't. He still needs a place to stay. The dream resolves itself in our agreeing that we will support one another wherever we may happen to be.

Becoming Aware

OF OLD PATTERNS

TIGHT NECK AND SHOULDERS. Clenched teeth. Shallow breathing. Knotted stomach. Self-defeating behaviors. Negative self-judgments. How do we develop such patterns? How can we change them if we're not aware of them and have no insight into their origins?

Fortunately, even if the mind has forgotten the origins, the body often remembers. During Rubenfeld Synergy sessions, most clients enter a state of deep relaxation in which their unconscious beliefs and long-buried memories can come to the surface.

In some of the stories that follow, memories emerge dramatically. In others, insights develop gradually over many sessions or between sessions. The authors of these stories include two former clients, as well as Synergists who have been in practice for anywhere from a few months to eighteen years.

Synopses

Listening for Metaphors. Three of Mary Jane's clients follow the metaphoric implications of their images—a window, a tired warrior, and stone walls. They discover old patterns and begin to change them.

Dream Body-Mapping. Gisèle's client Louise* has very little body awareness during her sessions. This begins to change when Gisèle has Louise draw images from a dream inside an outline drawing of Louise's own body.

Remembering Eddie. Janet's* memory of visiting her dying brother leads to her first-ever experience of anger at having been emotionally abandoned by her mother.

The Depths of Beliefs. Sonja writes about Rebecca,* a former client, whose forearm pain had forced her to abandon her career as a concert pianist. In a session Rebecca discovers and "erases" perfectionistic rules, which turn out to be connected to the pain.

Clues from Within. Linda writes about clients' images during sessions: Barbara's* images of trees support the healing of her shattered leg. Terry's* imaginary sprite-in-a-flower brings her peace. In a personal session of her own, Linda's images of playing cards reveal a previously unrecognized ambivalence.

Embodied Memories. Betty describes a session with her client J. R.* In a flashback J. R. connects his forty-year-old pattern of chronic, habitual tension to having felt responsible, at age three, for protecting his mother from harm.

Anchors Aweigh. Baffled by her inability to make progress toward her career goals, Rose discovers some self-defeating beliefs that have been blocking her.

Choosing a Partner. Renate reexperiences the abandonment she suffered as a child and discovers the roots of her pattern of choosing inappropriate romantic partners.

Sam's Story. Sam,* who has been seriously injured on a construction job, faces a major life crisis. His Synergist, Linda, describes a session in which Sam's memories from childhood help to bring release from chronic pain.

Tales My Left Leg Told Me. Joy writes about her three years of sessions with her Synergist, Lalitha, and some of the insights gleaned when Joy learned to "listen" to her left leg.

Learning the Conscious Good-bye. Margaret is troubled by certain aspects of the working relationship with her Synergist. After working through and resolving these issues, Margaret finally recognizes the roots of her longtime inability to resolve conflict without pain.

Listening for Metaphors

Mary Jane Hooper

When a client says she "feels split" or is "up against the wall" or "needs better boundaries," I often invite her to explore the image further, to see where it takes her. I'll ask, "What is it like to feel split?" or, "What does it feel like, up against the wall?" or, "Where in your body are you aware of a lack of boundaries?"

The images or figures of speech that prompt me to ask questions like these come from my clients as they lie on the table during a Rubenfeld Synergy session. Answering these questions requires my clients to go beyond their habitual ways of thinking and use their creative imaginations. Very often, as they explore an image to gain a deeper understanding of its metaphoric meaning, they are surprised by how precisely the metaphor captures their feelings and beliefs about themselves. Let me give you three examples from my practice.

DURING A SESSION with Lee, a school counselor, I placed my hands under her left shoulder and asked her to send a message to that shoulder or wait for an image from it. Lee said the image that came to her was a window; she was looking through a window at a group of people standing outside.

Not knowing what significance the window might have for Lee, I asked her, "Is the window open or closed?"

"It's closed," she answered. After a long pause she continued, "I feel a little guilty that I keep it closed."

As we continued to explore her image of the window, Lee discovered that she closed the window to set boundaries for herself. As a child she had felt responsible for her mother's happiness, and as a mother herself she now felt responsible for her children's happiness. Jessica, one of Lee's daughters, was blaming Lee for her own failed relationships with men. In response to these pressures, Lee would "shut the window." Lee realized that she would like to find a way to protect herself without shutting people out.

ANOTHER CLIENT, a young woman named Kathy, told me at the beginning of her first session that she felt her spirit was dying, that there was no passion in her life. She said she was exhausted from what felt to her like constant fighting. I could have asked her to say more about her dying spirit, her lack of passion, or her exhaustion. Any one of these might have led to a productive metaphor. But I was drawn to the energy with which she spoke about constant fighting and asked a question that would bring her attention to her body.

"What part of your body is doing the fighting?" I asked.

"My right side."

Later, when I placed my hand on her right hip, Kathy said she saw the image of an old Indian. "He looks defeated....He's my warrior."

"Where does your warrior reside in your body?" I continued.

"In my heart."

We began a dialogue with her warrior. Giving him a voice Kathy said, "I'm tired, I'm tired of fighting." She went on to describe some of the troubles she had experienced during the last few years. Then, after a long pause, she suddenly breathed a sigh and exclaimed, "I set a bird free...the bird is my spirit." I did not need to know by what path Kathy got from her warrior to her bird/spirit. The images and their metaphoric meaning were always hers, to use as she chose.

AT THE START of a session with Beth, a gifted artist, I slowly walked around her as she lay on the table and asked her what she was aware of in her body. She said that her left side felt free and her right side felt heavy. She described images of steel doors and stone walls and said she felt as if she were plowing her way through life and having to go through brick walls. Although she wanted to move forward in her life, she was in pain over the deteriorating health of her mother and the death of a child. She said she felt that all that kept her from falling apart were these walls—her body.

Images like these, with conflicting metaphoric meanings—walls as barriers, walls as safety—are often quite rich. Body metaphors don't have to make sense to be useful. In Beth's case it was their very lack of sense that made them useful. With one hand under Beth's right hip joint and one hand underneath her right knee, I began to trace the energy down her right leg and out the foot. As I did so she said it felt as if the walls were crumbling. Continuing our dialogue, Beth realized that the walls were not holding her life together; to the contrary, they were keeping her locked in fear from her painful past.

Exploring clients' metaphors does more than simply help them discover subtle emotional and behavioral patterns of which they have been unaware. As Lee, Kathy, and Beth got in touch with the meaning of their respective metaphors, they began to use the metaphors to explore alternatives—to transform their images into tools for creating positive change in their lives.

In subsequent sessions and in her life, Lee learned to open and close her window more freely. In the past she had felt guilty when saying no to her mother or her children. She could not make the voice of guilt go away entirely, but she could block it out by using the same image of closing the window. She had already used this metaphor to help her set clearer boundaries with her mother and daughter. Now she used it more consciously and in a slightly different way. She told Jessica that she was no longer willing to be blamed for Jessica's problems; Jessica had to take responsibility for herself. At the same time, Lee increased her own ability to make choices and to take better care of herself.

As Kathy explored the metaphor of her warrior, his role began to change. He no longer felt burdened by what he was carrying, but instead felt uplifted by it. Kathy developed a vibrant, positive image of her warrior as her true liberator. After several sessions she told me that she was experiencing renewed energy—a passion and sense of freedom in her life that was greater than she could remember having since she was a child.

After Beth began to talk about and to reexperience some of her past traumas, she saw a new image—a vortex. She saw the vortex as a tunnel or path through which she could release some of the fear and pain. As Beth began to use this new image her body began to relax, and as it did she was able to feel spaciousness and lightness where before she had felt walled in. After using the image of the vortex during sessions to practice "dissolving" steel doors and "tunneling through" brick walls, Beth began to use her vortex image outside of sessions, to make choices and to move forward in her life.

These are just a few examples of how the language of metaphor can lead clients to awareness and meaningful change. Exploring metaphors that "embody" their reality gives them opportunities to exercise their imaginations and open doors to new ways of looking at situations. Then, within the therapeutic environment, clients' experiences of self, others, and life can be more readily transformed.

Dream Body-Mapping

Gisèle Robert

*When Louise** first came to see me, her main complaint was chest pain that had bothered her for over ten years. Like several other Rubenfeld Synergy clients of mine, Louise found it difficult at first to notice subtle physical sensations or to "see" her body in her mind's eye. One day, after many sessions, she said that having some visual cues might help her in this regard.

During a subsequent session soon afterwards Louise said she wanted to explore a dream. I saw this as an opportunity to give her the visual cues she wanted because, as it happened, I had recently been studying Professor George W. Baylor's technique of dream body-mapping, which has the client draw dream symbols within an outline drawing of her body. When I told Louise about the technique, she said she loved to draw and became eager to try it.

I asked Louise to lie down on a large sheet of paper and I traced with a dark marker the contour of her outstretched body. Sitting on a chair a few feet from her, I then guided her in a short relaxation process with focused breathing, designed to facilitate an inner awareness. I next asked Louise to recount her dream to me, retelling it in the present tense and including details of the settings, characters, and principal objects, as well as the emotions she felt. When she had finished I asked Louise to sit up and begin to draw the various dream images within the outline of her body-map. I asked her to draw them intuitively, one symbol at a time. I invited her to visualize each symbol before drawing it, and to choose her colors carefully.

Louise sat on the floor and looked for a few minutes at the paper and box of colored pencils. Selecting a gray pencil, she drew the outline of a cat inside the contour of her left shoulder and arm. With a brown pencil she drew a different right arm and hand that crossed over her chest area, explaining as she worked that she wanted to hold the cat. She gave the cat a red tongue and a blue eye. As she added two blue eyes to her own face within the contour, she explained that the cat wanted to be seen. She continued to draw the cat by coloring his fur in the direction she would pet him. In the area of her stomach, she drew a brown bowl full of a white dessert. Louise took all the time she needed to finish her work and seemed to let the symbols emerge from inside her.

She did not pause between any of these first few drawings, but then seemed to have difficulty deciding where to place the next few symbols. I suggested that she scan her body with her hands as she visualized the next images. Touching her body slowly with her hands in a to-and-fro movement, she got a sense of where the images belonged on her body-map. She drew shutters on her chest and a group of people on her belly. She then wrote in black a sentence in her head: *«Peut-être pas dans cette vie»* (Maybe not in this life).

By now totally engaged in the process, Louise stood up to get a new sheet of paper. She placed the new sheet over the old and began to draw another cat. But—not wanting to separate the two cats—she returned to the first sheet and drew a second cat on her chest, lying outstretched and frozen, appearing from beneath the shutters.

All the while she drew, Louise expressed her emotions aloud and related some of the dream symbols to her current life situation. When she drew the first cat, she cried and connected the tears with her fear of losing something precious. Drawing the dessert bowl, Louise was moved and relieved by pointing out her nourishing relationship with her mother. She became sad while drawing the people on her belly, because she felt rejected by them. The shutters and the sentence intrigued her and the frozen cat shocked her, but she could not explain these symbols.

The drawing process took up most of the fifty-minute session, so I asked her to take her dream body-map home and keep it close to her until our next session. When Louise brought it back the following week we looked at it from the point of view of how it represented, on paper, the flow of her body's energy. And we began to discuss her dream symbols.

Louise described her head as a thoughtful witness that kept mute. She saw her left shoulder and arm as full of responsibility and needing to share the care. Her chest looked overloaded with blocked emotions. Her stomach seemed twisted by both resentfulness and forgiveness. Her belly was bursting with different duties, and her legs were empty and powerless. These observations and discoveries led to several sessions of Rubenfeld Synergy in which we dealt with these issues. In these sessions Louise was able to feel in her body some of the sensations and emotions she had expressed on paper.

The symbol that intrigued Louise the most was the frozen cat, so she started a dialogue with him. One by one the other symbols joined their conversation. Through this process Louise came to understand her loneliness and her poor self-esteem. Later she connected these feelings to her ongoing struggle to free herself from her mother's sadness.

As Louise lay on the table and talked about the symbols, and the symbols came alive and interacted and influenced one another, she felt more and more the flow of energy in her body. She started to feel her chest opening up and began to breathe differently. And her chest pains gradually decreased. Freedom from pain in this area freed her chest from old memories and helped her to make new life decisions. Now she was able to work better in her profession and to be more open with people in social situations.

As we continued to work together, Louise became much more confident in herself and in her ability to find answers deep within her own dreams, body, and life process. The informational components already present in her dreams were amplified by both dream body-mapping and Rubenfeld Synergy. The combination was responsible for much of Louise's healing and the healing of other clients with whom I have worked.

Remembering Eddie

Marita Bishop

Although blood tests showed that Janet's chronic liver disease was in remission, her body, mind, and spirit were faltering. Traditional counseling was helping her learn to cope with her illness, the deaths of family members, and emotional traumas from her youth. But when she first came to see me for massage therapy, she was suffering from terrible headaches, fatigue, anxiety, insomnia and depression.

After several massage sessions Janet's headaches had subsided and she was sleeping better. By this time I had advanced to the point in my Rubenfeld Synergy studies where I needed to procure "practice clients," people who were willing to let me practice my new skills without pay. When I invited Janet to be a practice client—I recall describing Rubenfeld Synergy to her as similar to "massage from the inside"—she readily accepted.

With each Rubenfeld Synergy session, Janet's anxiety diminished. In a paper for her college writing course Janet wrote: "I did not feel pressure to perform in any certain way. I began to accept my body and its messages as indicators of what was going on in my mind and spirit and with my emotions. I became aware of my body's posture and of tension in my muscles."

I would hold Janet's shoulder or hip between my hands while we talked of what she was experiencing. Sometimes she would "see" a vivid color and we would explore what the color meant to her. Other times she saw an object, a person, or a long-forgotten memory and we would explore that. Sometimes she saw nothing. As we talked I could feel her shoulder or hip gradually relax. This change did not come from an external massage; it came from within, as she released tensions that had been stored there during her lifetime.

Janet speculated about how the touch, body awareness, and recalling of memories helped her to recover from personal trauma. She said it reminded her of a mother caring for her infant—hands gently holding and cradling the baby, gentle words protecting her and accepting her for who she was. Not having received such soft, peaceful nurturing as a child, she called Rubenfeld Synergy her "second chance" to experience nurturing and to work through inner conflicts that had caused her muscles to "hold on" in the first place. She wrote in her paper, "New messages are sent to the brain and, with time and work, they 'reprogram' it so that the chronic tensions diminish or disappear."

After a few sessions Janet began to allow stored emotions to come forth. When she remembered a traumatic incident and allowed herself to feel the emotions related to it, she was able to work with the emotions and release the hold of that memory. I recall one session, in particular, when this occurred:

Janet slipped off her shoes and lay down on the massage table in my office. I asked her about her week and she told me about a headache that had lasted for two days. I asked her to notice how her body felt as she rested on the table. I cradled her head gently with my hands. When I touched her neck lightly, her head rolled only slightly from side to side. Now we were both aware of the tension in her neck.

Standing at her left side, I held her arm and moved one of my arms underneath her shoulder. "Bring your awareness to this area I am holding," I told her. "How does it feel?"

"Tense and tight," she replied.

"Is there any color or picture or image there?"

She told me about a very clear picture of her brother Eddie lying on a hospital gurney shortly after his car accident sixteen years ago, when she was fifteen. Soon, she began to experience waves of emotion. When I asked if she wanted to talk about it she replied, "I feel scared and very sad. Eddie has a broken neck, collapsed lungs, and a serious head injury."

Her story unfolded. Her mother, brothers and sisters were with them. After one look at Eddie, her mother headed for the door, telling Janet's sister Mandy, "Your brother is going to die."

As clients often do while reexperiencing old memories, Janet spoke as if the events were happening in the present. She continued, "I feel I should go with Mom, but I want to stay with my brothers and sisters. I don't want to leave Eddie alone."

I asked her, "How did you feel about your mother walking out and leaving you alone with Eddie?"

"Furious!" she blurted out.

I encouraged Janet to tell her mother how she felt.

"Wait, Mom," she cried, tears running down her cheeks. "We need help! Why can't you stay and help us? ...I am angry you're leaving. Why can't you think of us, too, and not just yourself?"

When Janet's sobbing subsided I brought her attention back to her shoulder, where my hands still rested. It felt very loose there; the tension had diminished greatly. When I asked how she felt she said, "Good; there is much less tension in my shoulder. I feel as if a great burden has been taken from me." She seemed much less anxious.

"Why do you think this memory was stored in this part of your body?" I asked her.

Her answer came quickly. "It was this part of Eddie's body that I held and touched when I visited him one month after the accident. He was coming out of a coma, and when I sat by his bed I stroked his shoulder and arm and talked to him. For a moment I saw his eyes open and he smiled a bit before sinking again into semiconsciousness. His small flicker of a smile encouraged me. It was painful to see Eddie like this, emaciated, rash-ridden, and covered with sores, but I wanted to be near him.... This was one of the last times I saw him alive."

Janet wrote about this session:

It was the first time I remembered this event, the first time as an adult that I saw what Mom did—and what she didn't do. Feeling angry was a new experience for me. When I was younger I learned to push anger down inside myself. That's how I survived. For the first time, I realized that Mom had abandoned us—not only at this event but at many events like it—and I cried....

Now, having shared this story, I can recognize the pain it created for so many years. I feel safe expressing anger when I am with my Synergist, who is warm, caring, and gentle.

With many succeeding sessions Janet discovered other connections between traumas and where they were stored in her body as pain or tension. And she wrote:

By bringing these painful memories into focus, I have gained an understanding of why I struggled with anxiety and depression. I used to layer new struggles on top of previous traumas. Now that these past issues have been resolved, I have more energy to deal with today's problems.

As my mood swings gradually lessen, I feel a greater sense of peace and clarity about who I am. No longer paralyzed by deep anxiety and fear, I am learning to see life as continual cycles that include tranquil moments to enjoy and rougher moments to work through. . . . Releasing the past frees my energy to try new things. I feel calmer and my confidence seems to be growing. When I make a mistake it's okay; I can learn from it. I am learning to accept myself as I am, as God made me.

The Depths of Beliefs

Sonja Contois

Healing work has been my life for over twenty years: Ericksonian Hypnotherapy, Neuro-Linguistic Programming, Applied Kinesiology, and more. These modalities were and are effective at easing my clients' physical and emotional pain—for a while. I have often wondered, "Why does the pain keep coming back?" and "Why is there pain in the first place?"

My instructors had little appreciation for these questions when I began asking them aloud. By November 1994 my growing frustration was outdistancing my growing kinesiology practice. My clients often had strong emotional reactions that intensified throughout a session; at times they were moved to tears as I pressed lightly on their neurolymphatic points. I had limited training to help me deal with these highly charged emotional responses, so I merely stayed with the clients without touching them further, and asked them to continue to experience their feelings. If words came to them, I was there to hear them. I felt that continuing to touch them, or moving to another point, would interrupt and negate what they were feeling.

I began to search for better means to support my clients in integrating their physical, emotional, mental, and spiritual lives. I wanted to learn a method that would enable them to bring about their own healing and balance. I found it in December of that year —while attending the weeklong Psychology of Health, Immunology, and Disease conference—at Ilana Rubenfeld's presentation of the Rubenfeld Synergy Method.

I was awed by the spirit of the work, the effectiveness of gentle touch, Ilana's use of humor, and the metaphors that emerged during her demonstration sessions. This was the method I'd been seeking. I applied for the next Rubenfeld Synergy Training Program, starting in January, a scant month away. Then I had a personal session with a Rubenfeld Synergist and got in touch with some of the memories that were stored in my body.

Almost three years have passed since then and my respect for the work keeps growing. My clients share my enthusiasm for Rubenfeld Synergy. Rebecca,* a young dancer, has given me permission to use her story.

Midway through our second session, lying on the massage table, Rebecca told me she had just become aware of an old, familiar pain in her forearm. I asked, "If that pain had a voice, what would it say to you?" The following dialogue ensued, with many long pauses for silent awareness and thought:

"'Be perfect,'" she answered. "'Be perfect.'" The pain spoke these words aloud, over and over, with increasing intensity and crispness, until it was barking a staccato, military command.

"Whose voice is that . . . giving you that rule, 'Be perfect'?" I asked.

"My piano instructor's."

"It's your piano teacher telling you to be perfect?"

"Yes."

"Are there other rules?"

"Yes," she said, adding, "'Win' and 'Look good.'"

"And whose rules are those?"

"They're her rules, from her rule book," she exclaimed with a slight overtone of indignity.

Rebecca and I explored the rules of childhood and those of adulthood. When I suggested that perhaps the childhood rules could be changed because she was now an adult, she uttered an excited "Wow!" She then decided that those first three rules needed erasing, since they continued to exert such negative power in her life.

At my invitation we conducted an experiment. Rebecca used a makeshift "eraser" to sweep down her arms, first one and then the other. Then she made wide sweeps through the air, erasing the three rules and their underlying power. She sighed deeply with every sweep; her body heaved with every sigh. Each rule took several sweeps before she felt it had disappeared.

When all the rules had vanished, I asked Rebecca if she would like to create a rule book of her own. She said yes. However, in order not to be trapped by rules, even those of her own making, she titled it *Rebecca's Erasable Rules.* She described the book, "opened" it, and began "writing." With wide sweeps of her hand, this time using her finger as a writing instrument, Rebecca entered her first two rules:

"Be free!" and "Have fun!" As the session came to a close the tension in her body melted like butter.

Rebecca also disclosed in this session that the forearm pain had driven her to abandon her previous career as a concert pianist. Although the pain had never gone away entirely, not until this session had Rebecca noticed a connection between emotional stress and flare-ups of the pain.

A week later Rebecca danced into my office for another session. With arms outstretched she said, "Driving home, the pain was gone except for a tiny area in my right forearm. When I listened to the pain, I knew it was my voice—laughing."

Recently I showed Rebecca the first draft of this story and asked for her permission to have it published. After reading it she made some comments. In reference to her exclamation of "Wow!" Rebecca said she realized that the old rules had always been just beneath the surface. But she had not understood consciously how much they were affecting her until that session, when she suddenly saw the whole picture.

She also said that the physical process of erasing old rules was so valuable that she has integrated it into her daily life. When, for example, her employer uses a certain tone of voice and phrases that clearly sound like his rules, she makes small erasing motions with her hand as a reminder that those rules are not hers.

As a Rubenfeld Synergist I see again and again how the body can literally accept and store as "truth" many outdated statements and ideas. I am awed by my clients' ability to become aware of their patterns and to release them—physically, emotionally, mentally, and spiritually—on their journey toward self-knowledge.

Clues from Within

Linda Stoffel

When she first came to see me, Barbara* was experiencing constant pain from injuries she had suffered in a car accident several months earlier. The pieces of her shattered left thighbone were held together with a metal plate and bolts. She was barely able to walk, even with the aid of a walker, and was discouraged by the lack of progress despite constant visits to physical therapists and doctors. A very active woman in her midfifties, she was suffering emotionally, as well as physically, from her inability to get around.

Early in our first Synergy session, as she was resting on the table, Barbara told me about an image that had just come to her. A scrawny, sticklike tree had another tree inside it that was full, lush, and beautiful. As we explored that imagery together in the session, she identified the stick tree as the façade she presents to the world and the wonderful tree inside as her true self, beautiful and whole. As she focused on the inside tree, it began to grow new buds and fruit. Animals made their homes in her tree; it was full of life. She began to feel physical sensations of warmth and energy all over, especially in the injured leg. This was the first time since the accident that she had felt anything but pain in her body, and she left this session feeling a sense of peace and joy.

By the start of our third session, Barbara's main concern was no longer the pain. Now she worried that she would never again be able to walk normally. She thought of herself as being in parts, not whole; the injured left leg depended on the healthy right leg to carry the weight and do all the work. Lying on the table she recalled her tree images and, becoming more aware of her legs, she reported seeing and feeling new tree images. Afterward, she wrote that her right leg was "very strong and straight, like a young sapling," and her left leg "like a grafting. All the pieces are put together. It doesn't look unhealthy as I thought it would. I had some fear that my leg wouldn't come back, but I don't have that [fear] anymore. I feel really good about this."

Barbara's positive images, coming spontaneously from within her, created positive feelings about herself and her leg. Exploring the images during our sessions helped her feel more relaxed and hopeful than she had in months. Seeing the possibility of someday being without pain supported her healing process over the next two years.

The power of imagery and its ability to foster healing has fascinated me for years, not only as a practitioner of Rubenfeld Synergy, but also as a client. In a session of my own several years ago, my Synergist asked me to send a message to my right hip while she was "sandwiching" it between her hands.

Immediately I saw an image of two hands dealing cards onto a pile of cards lying on a table. I was puzzled at first. Card playing held no significance for me. Then I became curious. When my Synergist asked me, "What about the cards?" I "saw" the jack of hearts. My thoughts moved to "gambling with my heart," then to "trusting my heart to someone else," and eventually to "I'm not yet willing to gamble with giving my heart to anyone."

At the time, I was struggling to understand my noncommittal attitude in a romantic relationship. My initial image proved to be a symbolic image of my emotional state. Its unusual content invited me to explore "the same old story" from a new perspective. The process of exploration, which required me to trust in it enough to temporarily suspend judgment, helped me to clarify my confusion.

Once in a while a client comes up with an image so extraordinary, detailed, and magical that it takes my breath away. This happened with Terry,* a creative and talented musician and songwriter. Our first two sessions had centered on her striving to be perfect, the tension and strain this striving put on her body, and her recent lack of creativity. In these sessions she had talked about feeling as though she had her feet in two worlds, between "a kind of middle-class conservatism and hippie idealism." She was struggling with the conflict between wanting to be both financially responsible and spontaneously creative. Here is a detailed excerpt from our third session together.

> I touch Terry's head and neck very lightly and ask what she is aware of in this moment. I notice that her body seems restless, unable to lie still. She stretches her legs and arms, yawns several times, and moves her hands as if trying to find a comfortable place for them. She doesn't tell me what

she's aware of so, after a while, I ask her which part of her body has the most energy.

"I don't know. The word *hands* comes into my mouth. My head is so...maybe...I don't know."

"What do you notice going on with your hands? See if there is an image that comes up when you focus on your hands."

After a pause she answers, "The only images coming up are the way my hands look. The first image is sort of a shape, sort of like this finger being raised up a little, like this." With her hands still lying on her chest, she raises her index finger.

I encourage her to give that finger a voice.

After another pause she reports, "The first thing that came to my mind was, 'It points the way' and the second thing was 'grace.'"

I repeat her words and put the two phrases together— "points the way to grace."

Terry points to her heart and says, "Something kind of did a tiny little bubble right here. I'm thinking it's like a whirlpool, something that kind of draws you down in, like a suction."

I ask Terry if she is willing to go into the whirlpool. She says yes. I notice her breath quieting and her body becoming more still. After a long pause Terry begins describing her image:

"Like a lily, very deep when it's closed. The petals are very long. The cup is very deep....It's open enough to go inside it....I'm sitting at the bottom of the cup. It has long golden stamens and a long golden pistil. It's like a womb, protection, a kind of refuge. I'm seeing an image of a tiny person in there, who I think is me."

I ask how the tiny person feels being in there.

"Like she's in sync with the vibes of the flower... giving her its grace, what she needs. A quiet place where she can be with herself. It's beautiful. It's soft. It's elegant. It smells nice."

I ask her how it is fulfilling her needs.

"A quiet place where she can be with herself....I need to make a place like that for myself to go into a lot." Terry describes the tiny "sprite" dwelling inside the flower as "very fresh and vibrant, with a face like a flower, sparkling blue-black eyes, and white, white skin."

Terry remains quiet for a long time, connecting to this sprite. Finally she whispers, "I think I've got it now. She's all the fine things that mean so much to me. If I devote myself to those fine things, the gross needs will take care of themselves somehow.... And it's a message for my hands... because they are the ones that play the piano... because they are graceful. My hands are why my parents bought me a piano, my entry into the world of things that are fine."

As we bring the session to a close, Terry says about her sprite, "Her face just beamed when I asked her if I could come down again to visit. She's always happy. That's how she related to me, with her hands. Her arms and hands were so graceful. It's as if she's my essence."

As I guide Terry to a sitting position, both of us have tears in our eyes. I am amazed by how much different she looks now from when she arrived. Her face is radiant and vibrant. Her head is up; her shoulders are comfortably dropped; her body is completely relaxed.

We sit quietly for a while, not wanting to disturb the

moment or Terry's connection to the deep, quiet, nourishing place she has found within herself, to which she can return whenever she chooses.

I have witnessed many such instances of images that accurately and creatively reveal emotions and unconscious beliefs. Not limited by the rules of logic, imagery can bypass habitual mental blocks and tap into the entire wealth of body wisdom, making it available for exploration and personal growth.

Embodied Memories

Betty Esthelle

I am fascinated by the way the Rubenfeld Synergy Method encourages long-held, "embodied" experiences to surface into consciousness. Once clients feel safe enough in both the therapeutic relationship and their own bodies, they begin to let go of habitual tensions. Let me give you an example of this from many years ago:

> J. R.* is a well-educated, successful psychotherapist who has been in private practice for nine years. Having completed his therapy with a Gestalt practitioner, he comes to see me in order to explore his constant fear and tension. This is J. R.'s sixth session.
>
> As J. R. settles onto the table, I am aware of the seemingly random, small, involuntary movements of his wrists,

feet, and head that have been evident in his previous sessions. These tiny "tics" remind me of flicking off an annoying insect. We have previously determined the movements to be so small as to be out of his awareness. I notice his shallow breathing and am surprised that even though this man sings, he does not breathe into his belly.

I invite J. R. to breathe into his lower belly. As he does so J. R. begins to relax and to visualize and embody the ideas of softening, lengthening, and widening that we have practiced in previous sessions. His breathing gradually deepens until his belly moves smoothly with each inhalation and exhalation. The expression on his face softens and he looks peaceful and contemplative. I notice that his tics have stopped.

As the session proceeds, largely in silence, J. R. comments that his fear is related somehow to his mother. After another long silence he reports that it is his mother's fear he's feeling. This revelation is colored with waves of inadequacy followed by powerful anger. When his red face and growling cries have subsided, he takes several deep and quieting belly breaths. Then he begins to breathe more deeply, at the level of the solar plexus,[1] which is considered the center of the emotions in many Eastern healing arts. J. R. weeps quietly and tells me of his grief and sadness. He thanks me for the support he feels from my hands, which have been resting beneath his back much of the time.

Later, as the session comes to a close, J. R. says that he feels relaxed for the first time he can remember in a long time. His joy is apparent as he dances and sings around the room. Then he shares with me part of what he experienced

---

[1] A dense network of nerves located in the abdomen behind the stomach and in front of the aorta.

during the session, when he remembered feeling responsible for protecting his fearful mother.

I felt my mother's fears. I didn't even know why she was afraid. She didn't tell me. Perhaps she didn't even know herself. I looked and looked. I looked everywhere for some monster, some dreadful danger. I looked to find that terrible threat.

And I got ready....I got ready to fight for my mother. I loved her. She was my life, my identity....My arms got ready, the muscles about to strike. My legs got ready, tense thighs, knees pulled up, feet ready to spring into action. My neck and my eyes were searching for that enemy. My stomach muscles tightened to protect my innards in the coming battle. Even my jaw got ready, ready to snarl with ferocity. My neck strengthened like steel to hold my head....I was only three years old and I would protect my mother.

I never found that enemy....I am still prepared for that fight....Until now, I never remembered. I couldn't relax and I didn't know why....I got ready for that battle forty years ago.

This session of J. R.'s, although unusually dramatic, is typical of the power of the unconscious to withhold information somewhere in the body until the client feels safe and supported enough for that information to reveal itself.

Anchors Aweigh

Rose M. Andrzejewski

It was a dark day in February. I was sitting on one of those uncomfortable plastic chairs at La Guardia Airport, waiting for my flight to Buffalo to visit my mother, who had undergone major surgery the week before. I had taken this Sunday off from rehearsals for a regional theater production of *Evita* to be with my mother when her diagnosis came down. My boyfriend had just broken up with me. My singing and dancing mentor was gravely ill. Commuting between temp jobs, production assignments, and voice lessons in Manhattan and rehearsals in Connecticut was taking its toll on me. I was exhausted.

I slumped in the chair as I realized that all my efforts were not bringing me closer to realizing my dreams—of singing on Broadway and being financially independent. Now, worrying about my mother's diagnosis, it was all I could do not to fall apart. I was running hard, but in too many different directions. I decided right then to start doing things differently.

When I returned from Buffalo, I began to look into bodywork and counseling. I gained some insight into a pattern I had not been aware of—starting one project after another and dropping each one before it had a chance to bear fruit. I would start each new venture with enthusiasm and energy, but sooner or later I would lose steam and let the project fade away. Recognizing this pattern did not help me change it. I continued searching for a more effective modality.

I was drawn to Rubenfeld Synergy because of Ilana's background as a musician. Wondering if a healing approach developed by a musician might work better for me than some of the others I'd tried, I began having sessions with a Synergist who had been a dancer before becoming a counselor. I took to the work at once and soon decided to accelerate my personal growth by taking the Rubenfeld Synergy Training. I remember one session in particular that brought me to a new level of self-knowledge.

> Lying on the table, I kept thinking to myself how good it felt not to have to do anything, and just to be. As Diane, my Synergist, gently touched my head, I noticed a lot of tightness and tension in my body.
>
> Diane: What are you noticing?
> Rose: I notice that my left leg and foot feel connected to the table and my right leg and foot are going out to the side. I feel off-balance.
> D: Do you have an image or message for your left leg?
> R: It's an anchor. It feels glued to the table. It is very solid and has a lot of strength.
> D: What about your right leg?

R: My right leg feels as if it's going in many different directions.

As I said this, my right hand made a back-and-forth motion.

D: What is that hand motion about?
R: It represents the chaos in my life.

As I thought about what I had just said, I began to cry intensely. I experienced a rush of energy through my pelvis and legs as I let go of some of the tightness there. I was suddenly aware that I could no longer run away from my problems.

Gradually my crying subsided and there was silence. As I allowed myself to be with the silence, a lot of emotions came up. I tried to ignore them but couldn't hold them back. A flood of feelings came pouring out of me. I started crying even harder about all the energy I had wasted going in so many directions without getting closer to my goals. I felt Diane's presence and sensed that she understood the pain and sadness I was experiencing. She waited for my tears to pass.

D: Rose, the anchor of a ship comes up when the ship goes out to sea.

I was perplexed by this. I had always thought of anchors as staying in the ocean and providing support and strength. The possibility that my anchor might come up scared me.

D: What would it be like to move forward?
R: Scary!

This was the first time I had ever realized that I was afraid of moving forward. But my body's signals were clear. My left side, my "anchor," was afraid to move anywhere and my right side went in many directions. Either side, by itself, was enough to explain my not moving forward toward my goals. The combination made it doubly impossible. I felt safer keeping my anchor in the ocean even though it meant going nowhere. But what was I afraid of?

After many more sessions I discovered that I was afraid of the consequences of becoming visible—for example, being compared to others, feeling awkward when receiving acknowledgment for my work, having to live up to higher expectations, maybe even being "lonely at the top." Each time I became aware of a fear during a session I would face it squarely and feel it crumble, only to discover a new layer of fear underneath. Gradually, by working through the layers, I was able to lay these fears to rest.

My original focus on personal growth evolved into a desire to share my healing with others by practicing Rubenfeld Synergy professionally. I faced a lot of challenges along the way and—of course!—at times thought about not continuing with the program. This time, though, I asked for help and worked through my inner conflicts instead of changing directions midcourse.

I am now ready to be seen and recognized, both as a Certified Rubenfeld Synergist and as a singer. I take concrete steps toward my personal and professional goals, knowing that it will take time, as well as hard work, to reach them. I'm not in a hurry anymore. I've slowed down enough to take pleasure in developing my practice and to enjoy the process of putting my cabaret act together.

For me the turning point was that session when I began to understand my need to run. By facing my fears I have found a new sense of freedom and peace.

Choosing a Partner

Renate Novak

In my late thirties, I became increasingly aware of the fact that my second marriage was just not working, and that it was time to do something about it. I was doing well in other areas in my life. I loved being a mother and was successful in my work, but how to be happy in a long-term romantic relationship was a mystery to me. It was fun and easy to get swept up in the beginning stages of falling in love. However, as I had experienced several times, the longer a relationship continued, the more the excitement would fade, until eventually I was left feeling misunderstood, unappreciated, and used. This is what was happening with my husband and me. No matter what I tried to do to improve the relationship, I ended up feeling sad and frustrated. I was tired of repeating this pattern.

A casual acquaintance, Jeanne Reock, told me she was studying Rubenfeld Synergy, a type of body-centered psychotherapy. She needed people to practice with for ten sessions[1] and asked if I was interested. Never having tried any kind of psychotherapy, I was curious and accepted her offer.

I especially remember the first few sessions because of their powerful effect on my body and sense of myself. While gently touching or holding my head, my shoulder, or some other part of my body, Jeanne would ask me to bring my attention to that area—to notice any sensations I was feeling and exactly where I felt them. Since I was not suffering from any physical pain, it often took me a few moments to locate a sensation.

In one early session, I noticed a subtle pressure in my chest and told Jeanne about it. She asked me what that pressure in my chest might say if it had a voice. Out of that question a "conversation" developed between me and the sensation. Before long I was connected to a hurtful memory from my childhood—the sadness of being left alone with an old grandmother who didn't love me. (My mother, who had never married, was away at work all day until late at night; I never knew my father.) The feelings of sadness and the pain in my chest grew stronger until they were almost unbearable, seeming to crush my chest. The slight pressure I had noticed there earlier had been only an indication of the strong emotions buried for many years. Feelings of being unloved and deeply lonely surfaced from inside my body. These were not distant, colorless memories of my childhood; I felt as if I were right there reliving them. I experienced them with my whole being and connected deeply with myself as that child.

In my sessions, when I experienced painful memories, I would release the associated feelings through tears and breath. It was like letting go of a trapped ghost.

---

[1] Practice clients can be seen for only a limited number of sessions.

With Jeanne's guidance I examined other situations that had made a strong impact on my life. Over the course of several sessions I came to see that, when it came to intimate relationships, I was still living my life out of my childhood experiences. In order not to feel unloved, misunderstood, and lonely, I had accepted anyone who wanted me, without checking to see if there was a basis for a good relationship. If a man let me know that he liked me and wanted to be with me, that was enough for me—for a while, at least, until it inevitably became clear how unsuited we were for one another.

In the sessions with Jeanne I came to understand that I had always deserved love, that I had been a lovable little child, and that the way I had been treated had distorted how I felt about myself. A new sense of appreciation for myself gradually replaced the sadness and self-pity. As I started to value myself more, I wanted to have people around me who loved me and treated me well. I began to see that my second husband was not the kind of man the new, more aware "I" wanted to be with. Staying in the marriage to avoid being alone didn't make sense to me anymore.

Soon after my last session with Jeanne, my husband and I decided to separate. I lived happily on my own with my son for the next three years and learned to recognize the experience of being respected and honored. I grew to like myself and feel at peace with myself. Delighting in getting to know myself in a whole new way, I felt happy and free. I am now in a very conscious relationship with a man who loves me and values me. We communicate well and understand each other. I've come a long way from feeling used, unappreciated, and misunderstood.

Sam's Story

Linda Thomas

Sam and I have worked as a healing "team" for over a year. I see him twice a week. His life has been that of giver, toiler, ambulance corps volunteer, flea market entrepreneur, and horticultural genius. Apple, peach, and berry pie baker—from his own orchards—he is also a friend of and gardener for an elderly local widow who has a roadside vegetable stand. He is snowplower and clam and oyster shell shucker for group events in town. Sam loves to go dancing. He has won many a country-western dance contest and he wears boots that his singing idols would admire.

In wintertime, when Sam regularly visits his mother's grave in the town cemetery, he notices which graves have been neglected and creates wreaths from his woodlands for them. He lays them with his stiff, callused hands and in his hearty, generous, and determined spirit. Sam is an unsung hero.

Now in his fifties, Sam has toiled since he was six years old and his father put him to work daily in his lawn care business. His very identity is only secure when he can work and give. If working hard is his identity, and dancing is, according to Sam, his "true calling," what will become of him if he is robbed of these two capabilities? That is the question that brought Sam to his life crisis and to his appointments with me for Rubenfeld Synergy.

In 1993, while doing roadwork with heavy equipment, Sam was hit in the back with a load of steel. The list of his surgeries and medical procedures since then creates a file thick enough to awe any physician and to stop a lesser human spirit dead in his tracks. There have been multiple spinal surgeries; his stomach ruptured and was fastened with mesh; some bowel has been removed; his heart is taxed from the physical labor and emotional heartache.

Since the road accident Sam's lifestyle has changed dramatically. Confined by chronic pain and medical interventions, Sam grieves the loss of his former physical strength and active lifestyle. Dancing, gardening, and volunteering—the great pleasures in his life—are no longer available to him. And most painful of all, his wife of many years, whom he loves deeply, has abandoned him for a healthier partner.

I have been seeing Sam around issues of depression and loss. During this past year Sam had to face a fourth spinal surgery. After an exhaustive search for relief from his physical pain, brought on by scar tissue that compressed spinal nerves, he found the prize neurosurgeon in the state. She pulled no punches. She would perform surgery if Sam accepted the risks: He could die; he could be permanently paralyzed; or he could come out of it with movement and, after recovery, without pain. Sam's only thought was, "It's worth the risk; I want my life back. Let's do it."

Sam and I have many Rubenfeld Synergy sessions in preparation for the surgery, including some challenging work about giving up control and allowing loving care to come into his heart for once in his life. Deeply afraid to take a chance on letting love in, Sam has played it safe all his life by being the giver. Our sessions allow us both to notice Sam's body's barrier against receiving and to discover his more deeply buried longing to feel supported.

As the date of the operation approaches, I make the decision to go the hospital and see Sam through the surgery. Since Sam has no family and is used to facing things alone, he becomes afraid. This provides a rich ground for our therapeutic work. I obtain permission from the hospital staff to be with Sam in the holding room and we do a Rubenfeld Synergy session just moments before the surgery. The staff watch with curiosity and much respect. Sam looks peacefully at me as he is wheeled off.

Prayers fill my time outside the operating room, and when the grueling six-and-a-half hour surgery is completed, I go to the recovery room and find this beautiful human being looking radiant. "My toes wiggle!" he beams.

It is now nine weeks later. As I look at Sam's feet in soft brown socks resting on my Synergy table, he tells me he has recovered much movement and has not experienced the old pain in his hip and leg at the site of the injury. He tells me he feels new life wanting to come into his body and he wants to move forward with it.

In characteristic "Sam style" he berates himself for not working today. He just "took the day off" and rested before coming to his session. He says he will make up for his "lazy attitude" by planting a shipment of new seedlings on his property tomorrow—fifteen hundred of them!

During the session we focus on his right shoulder, which has always done the lion's share of physical labor. Sam's hands and arms are, as usual, stiff and "held" as though they must always be ready for work and dare not relax. Although he sometimes experiences acute pain, his right shoulder has only the usual dull ache.

Linda: Sam, you know, it's okay to take a day off. No harm done.

Sam: Yeah, well, wait 'til tomorrow. I hate myself when I do this.

L: (with one hand supporting his right shoulder from underneath and the other gently cradling the top of it) Sam, bring your awareness to this shoulder. This shoulder is tired...so tired.

S: Well, it ain't seen nothing yet!

L: "Oh, Sam!" says your shoulder, "I'm really tired and I need you to listen to me. Please, Sam."

S: (Sam's shoulder lets go a bit, then tightens again. Sam is deep in reflection.) I *hate* it when someone says to me, "(in a mocking tone) Well, what did you do today?" *Like I don't work!*

L: That's right. You deserve a break...so tell your shoulder it's okay to be tired for one day.

S: Ha! If you think you hurt now, just wait 'til tomorrow.

L: I'll show you!

S: (grinning, eyes closed) You got it!

Sam's shoulder and upper back under my hands feel locked and completely silent. I note that his head is also locked straight on top of his neck, seeming to make no engagement with the rest of his body, and I imagine that his head might be rejecting a relationship with his shoulder.

I gently remove my hands and walk over to Sam's left shoulder, recalling that Sam writes with his left hand even though he does everything else with his right hand. I silently invite the left shoulder to release any burden it chooses. The left shoulder and arm become noticeably softer. I return to the right side and once again cradle it. (Sam likes the warmth of the touch and has allowed himself this pleasure since we first started working together. After our first session he had commented that the warmth was unbelievable and "like magic.") So we just stay with the warmth, waiting in silence and mutual listening. After a while my mind flashes to young Sam, and I become curious.

Linda: (pondering) Sam, what did your dad used to say to you when you were a kid and you wanted to go play like the other kids?

Sam: He'd say, Didn't I want to work? Did I want to be a shiftless, lazy bum?

L: How do you feel when you hear him saying that?

S: Terrible...ashamed... (The shoulder blade tenses more beneath my hands.)

L: What do you wish your dad would have said?

S: (long silence)

L: I mean, say you could write the script. What words would you give to him?

S: (with gravity and solemnity) "You done a good job." (Opening his eyes and looking back at me behind him.) Because he never said that, either. (Closes his eyes.) So, let's see, "You done a good job. Take the day off. No need to kill yourself...." Something light like that.

This is one of those stunningly beautiful moments in therapy when I catch my breath and say to myself, "Thank you, God." We continue to wait in silence.

L: (softly and respectfully) Wow, that's wonderful. Okay.

So, Sam, I want you to turn your head toward your right shoulder now.

S: (turns his head toward his right shoulder)

L: Now say that to your right shoulder, Sam.

S: (eyes fly wide open; looks up at me and grins) Oh, you're good!

L: (grinning back, knowing how Sam likes to scrap. I feel very solid in our bond.)

S: (begins to laugh and shake; his belly bounces)

L: Go ahead…close your eyes…go inside…keep with your body's experience. That's right. Tell your right shoulder what you always wanted to hear.

S: (still laughing) What was it? I forgot!

L: Go back and get it; it came from you. Tell me.

S: (takes a big, slow breath and releases it noisily; gets serious, then soft-spoken) You did a good job. (Blows his breath out with great release through puffed cheeks.)

L: Yeah. And I think there's even more.

S: You did a good job. Take the day off.

L: Yeah, there it is. Just breathe that in, Sam. Let your shoulder know. You finished? Or is there more?

S: Yeah. No need to kill yourself. (Much letting go, much deep breathing. Sam's neck is very soft and moves freely when I roll his head gently from side to side. Sam is breathing deeply and peacefully.)

L: (hands cradling Sam's right shoulder) Your shoulder hears you, Sam. (Long pause, listening in silence.) It's remembering those teenage years when you wanted to say to your dad, "I'm going to the Finnigan place for wood chips." You know, Sam, where Mary worked? And you two fell in love? Well, you wanted to say,

"Dad, I'm going to get wood chips, and I'll be just a little late!"

S: (big belly laugh and more shoulder contact with my
hands) Boy, you got that right! (Tears roll down Sam's
face. Sam has a fabulous sense of humor. Laughter is a
major release for Sam.)

L: I'm just listening to you and your body. Sounds to me
like *you* got it right.

We conclude the session with Sam's noticing his body's response
to the messages he had previously rejected: "You did a good job."
"Take the day off." "No need to kill yourself." Sam also recognizes
a paradox in himself: "I can't control everything by working and
giving, yet my heart is the biggest part of me."

As Sam moves forward along his life's journey, with deeper
self-recognition, I know he will bring to everything he does his
astonishingly bright life spirit, his generous heart, his gift for
laughter, his determination to dance again, and—especially—the
new life he feels coming in. I just have this feeling that he will be
fine.

Tales My Left Leg Told Me

Joy Gates

When I began working with Rubenfeld Synergist Lalitha Devi in 1993, I had already delved into many personal growth strategies, participated in individual and group Transactional Analysis, and studied the writings of innovators in the field of psychology. In short, I was not a virgin to the realm of inner work.

With Lalitha I learned practical life skills that added depth to what I had learned intellectually. We worked together in individual sessions about twice a month for almost three years until I moved out of state.

At the start of each session, I would sink into the comfortable couch in Lalitha's small office and fill her in on the events of my life since the last time. Sometimes we worked on a meaningful dream, and I would act out the various roles. Sometimes I just poured my heart out about my work or my marriage. But no matter what I talked about initially, the heart of the session started when I climbed onto the bodywork table, lay down, relaxed, and got in touch with my body and the feelings I held there so deeply.

Attending to my bodily energies, dialoguing with and helping my body to express deeply held experience, worked well for me. Lalitha would begin by gently moving my head, moving my arms and legs up and down and flexing them slowly, or pressing on my back muscles. I would gradually relax and calm my mental buzz. This body-centeredness always took me beyond my active mind into a realm new to me, where impressions and feelings rose whole into my awareness, bypassing my usual judgments. Like strange and exotic luminous fish slowly rising to the surface of deep, dark water, these feeling-communications were amazingly energizing to me.

Descriptions of the following two sessions are excerpted from the journal I kept at the time. In these sessions, I experienced my left leg in ways that allowed me to reconnect with parts of myself that I had disowned early in life.

September 1994

I am already on the bodywork table when I remark, "I think that the reduced flexibility in my left leg is just the way it's made and not something I'm imposing on it." As I speak, my leg develops a cramp—first in a toe, then in the foot as well, and finally extending up the calf to the knee. "Ow!" I yelp. "I've got a cramp in my leg! Maybe I'm holding something emotional in this leg after all."

"What does your left leg want to say?" Lalitha asks me.

"I'm not ready yet to give it voice. I'm not ready." I feel stubborn, resistant—no nice, cooperative, good little girl here

now. Gradually the cramping eases as Lalitha cradles the leg, moving it gently. After a while I am willing to give voice to it. I open my mouth, only to discover that my leg is stiffly resisting my appeal for words. I tell Lalitha, "I need to allow words gradually. I can't rush this." The leg feels better. I can sense energy flowing, a column of energy connecting with the torso.

"I can tell you this much," I say. "The feelings held in the leg seem to relate to sorrow and loneliness, anger and pain." My voice thickens with emotion. "I think that maybe my leg got caught in a viselike crack when I was a baby—maybe in my crib. I feel that it happened before I could talk and, perhaps, that stiffness and wordless suffering and being alone with my pain entered into my experience this way." I feel tired now, as if I've lifted weights. I resolve to work at home with my left leg, giving it voice.

The next day my left leg and I cooperate on this poem:

THE TALE MY LEFT LEG TOLD ME

Darkness looms over my speechless existence.
Pain and ignorance allow no end
to the dull pressure of duration.
I am durable and silent,
but do not mistake that for acceptance.
Within, I mourn, I rage and cry through the night
trapped in my restraints,
which are no less binding
because they cannot be seen.
At the heart of my reflection
there is darkness.
In the depths of my confession

there are no words.
I have dared to tell this tale
because it is the only door marked "Exit"
and I want my suffering to speak.
I need the words to give shape and form,
to clarify the nameless darkness,
amorphous in the realm of wordlessness.
Opening silently into the pain,
softly I speak at last.

November 1995

Lalitha is moving my feet gently back and forth—first my left foot, then my right foot. I notice my effort to keep up with her and I ask myself, "What is she looking for? Does my foot move enough? The left foot is not moving as much as the right! What could this mean? What should I do?" As I become aware of my silent chatter I realize that it serves as a protection, a shield. I begin to feel lonely and cut off, isolated by my constant chatter.

As I share these thoughts with Lalitha, I realize that my "little one"—myself as a child—really needs to know what people want from her or else she can be hurt. Tears well up in my eyes and compassion fills my heart for this frightened, eager-to-please-and-be-loved part of me.

"Why don't you talk to this little child?" Lalitha suggests.

When my throat is no longer tight I say, "Know this, Little One. You are not alone. You have help now, and everything isn't all up to you anymore. I am here to help now and to be your friend." Lalitha gently touches my left foot.

I become aware of an increasing integration of my "little girl" with other members of my "inner zoo"—the angry rebel, the efficient do-gooder, the head-tripper. I feel more embodied, too, enjoying a growing appreciation of spaciousness, of broad land, wide waters, and clear sky, and of thoughts and feelings that feel less crowded and dense, lighter and airier. Telling Lalitha this, I pause. "I really think this spaciousness is akin to spirit. I feel a deepening connection with my greater essence."

Since I left New York I have continued to benefit from the process we began in those sessions, as I use my new skills like fine, sturdy carpenter's tools. I am thriving now, not just surviving. I have learned to value my body and to take time every day to listen to my body's messages. And I have found a few other people who are receptive to hearing my truth. I see myself mirrored back by them and feel heard, seen, and validated. Telling my story—so that others may know they are not alone in their strangeness—is one aspect of my thriving.

As my left leg has said, "I have dared to tell this tale because it is the only door marked 'Exit.'"

Learning the Conscious Good-bye

Margaret A. Healy

One of my most valuable experiences with the Rubenfeld Synergy Method involved, perhaps surprisingly, the process of ending my work with Claudia,* my first Synergist.

I found Claudia by calling the Rubenfeld Center in New York. In our initial session I felt very attracted to her attention to detail and her respectful, noninvasive style. During subsequent sessions I found that Claudia was willing to meet me wherever I was emotionally and to simply be with me without judgment. I came to trust her more than any therapist I had worked with before. I became committed to ongoing work with her and, over time, we developed a strong therapeutic relationship.

Feeling certain that Rubenfeld Synergy was right for me—professionally as well as personally—I applied for the upcoming training. When it began, Claudia became my official "at-home" Synergist. By then we had been working together for almost two years. I continued to see her regularly except for the weeks of training in Manhattan.

During those training modules I had sessions with other Synergists, who were on the training faculty. Having this chance to experience another Synergist's style piqued my curiosity and I soon began to wonder what it would be like to work with a different Synergist back home. I felt a little guilty about thinking such "disloyal" thoughts, so whenever I caught myself in one of these fantasies, I would shake it off and tell myself that I didn't need to see someone else; I was doing fine with Claudia. Maybe our working relationship wasn't exactly perfect, but it would be counterproductive for me to switch to someone else and start the long process of learning to trust a new person.

A few months later, after another training module, the fantasies were still with me and I realized that they were based on more than just curiosity. I thought they might stem from some discomfort I felt in certain aspects of my working relationship with Claudia. It was very hard for me to identify those aspects and to find words to describe my experience of them. Yet after much soul-searching I identified two troubling situations.

One of these had to do with my response to certain memories that I accessed during Rubenfeld Synergy sessions. When each memory of early-childhood abuse surfaced, I would relive it in the present until I became overwhelmed by fear of physical attack. I sometimes felt pain in my stomach and back, as if I were actually being attacked. When this happened I would slide off the table onto the floor and scoot around the room in an attempt to get away from the pain. By the end of the session, I would be thoroughly exhausted, physically as well as emotionally.

Claudia would ask me what I needed in order to feel safe

enough to move through these memories, but I did not know how to answer her. These episodes kept recurring until I realized that, although I wanted to *get* on the table in order to go inside and confront my demons, I no longer wanted to *be* on the table.

The second situation that made me uncomfortable was bumping into Claudia at social events. We lived in the same town and knew some of the same people, so this was bound to happen. The problem was that in my sessions with Claudia, I often showed a very vulnerable side of myself, so that the first time I saw her at a social event I felt confused and awkward, not knowing how to interact with her in this new and different setting. I became self-conscious and retreated inside myself. Unable to be spontaneous, I did not enjoy myself as much as I usually did. The second time we both showed up at an event, I felt the same discomfort and realized that I would not be able to do my therapeutic work if I kept seeing Claudia socially.

When I told Claudia of my discomfort she helped me explore my deep upset about the possibility that our social circles might overlap again, and we came to an agreement about how to deal with the situation. We decided that whenever there was any doubt about which of us would be attending a particular social gathering, we would call and check it out with one another. In doing so we hoped to avoid any further blurring of the therapeutic boundary between Synergist and client.

This agreement worked well until one Friday night, when I was given the evening off—a rare occurrence. At the last minute I went to the circle dances I almost always missed on account of work. It didn't occur to me that Claudia, who knew I worked every Friday, might be there, too. When I saw her I instantly felt uneasy. I knew from our previous unexpected meetings at circle dances that she would try to minimize my distress by going out of her way not to be partnered with me. I also imagined that her efforts to lessen my discomfort might diminish her enjoyment of the evening. I felt terrible about my mistake and was certain that Claudia would be as annoyed with me as I was with myself.

My upset over this situation so exacerbated my general anxiety about going for sessions that I let several weeks go by without making an appointment. During this break, a week of Rubenfeld Synergy training provided me with some insight into the impasse I had reached. I did not get on the table in any of my personal sessions during that training week; I sat on the floor instead. In one particular session with Peggy, my Synergist for that week, I had a breakthrough.

In that session, when I experienced my usual overwhelming anxiety I began my familiar pattern of scooting around the floor. I kept moving away from Peggy and said over and over, in a very young voice, "I'm afraid of being touched" and "I don't want to get on the table." Peggy scooted around after me, staying very close during the entire session. Sitting next to me she would put her hands very gently on my feet or on my hands, and I would relax slightly for a moment or two. I didn't want to move away from Peggy—in fact, I wanted to be soothed by her—but the anxiety kept kicking in, and I felt compelled to move away each time. Peggy didn't give up, though, and each contact brought me a little more calm to displace the fear. My anxiety gradually lessened, and by the end of the session I was calm enough that I held still and rest for a few minutes while Peggy kept her hands on my feet.

I didn't see this session as a breakthrough until three days later, during a discussion with my training advisor. As we talked, I saw that each time Peggy had touched me, I had maintained the contact a little longer before moving away. In response to Peggy's contact, my fear had gradually decreased instead of increasing as I might have expected. Amazed, in retrospect, that I had not spiraled off into physical pain, I finally saw that my real, ongoing fear was not of being touched, but of being hurt.

I had learned this distinction during the session—not from Peggy's words, but rather from her touch and the intention behind it. Despite my fears and mental paralysis, *my body* had understood from her touch that I was with her in the present moment and that she was not going to hurt me. Being touched by Peggy *while* I was in that anxious state had helped me distinguish present reality from past memories—enough so I could calm down. My body had understood the message in her touch immediately; three days later I found words to describe my body's experience and understand it in a conscious way.

As I continued to reflect on the session with Peggy, I came to believe that what was missing from my sessions with Claudia was her touching me in a way that would allow me to learn that I was not being hurt in the present moment. I imagined that Claudia's initial instinct, whenever I was experiencing physical pain, might have been to use touch for this purpose, and that she chose not to touch me only out of respect for my unspoken signals to stay away, especially my scooting away from her. With neither of us knowing exactly what I needed in order to feel safe, I was drowning in pain and afraid to have sessions. The session with Peggy gave me the answer to Claudia's question: What did I need in order to feel safe enough in the present to move through painful memories? I needed to be grounded through touch.

Back home after that training week, I called Claudia and scheduled a session that would focus on aspects of our working relationship. I made it clear that I would sit on the floor and not get on the table. As the day of our session approached, I panicked: Would Claudia be offended when I told her what was bothering me? Would she would break off contact with me?

Within minutes of beginning the session, however, I found that my fears were completely unwarranted. When I spoke apologetically about showing up at the circle dances, Claudia said it was not important *how* it had happened, only that it *had* happened, and that what needed to be addressed were my upset feelings. When I told her about my recent breakthrough session with Peggy, she was happy to hear about my new insights. I asked Claudia if, during the sessions in which I kept scooting away from her, she had ever felt torn between wanting to ground me in the present by touching me and wanting to respect my body's cues not to touch me. She said that had been her dilemma exactly, and that she had chosen not to touch me in order to avoid the risk of retraumatizing me.

Claudia was eager to hear my thoughts, feelings, and ideas so that she could help me find a way to move through the impasse and proceed with my personal work. She didn't get defensive when I expressed my feelings completely about both situations. She encouraged me to decide for myself what course of action to take, whether that meant adjusting our working relationship or ending it. It was clear to me that Claudia wanted only what was best for me and that she would not try to influence my decision. Being given this freedom to choose for myself brought home to me my right, as a client, to be heard without being judged, and to be responded to without having my feelings dismissed as wrong or invalid. I left this session feeling relieved and empowered.

In subsequent "talk-only" sessions, Claudia and I continued to examine the complex layers of our relationship, especially those aspects with which I was uncomfortable. We considered various ways of modifying our working relationship, and when we discussed the option of ending our work, Claudia offered to help me find a new Synergist if I decided to go that route.

Having open communication like this in a therapeutic relationship was new to me, and very surprising. I experimented with this new freedom and found that, with each session, I increased my ability to trust myself, reclaim my voice, and speak honestly about my experience. After three sessions, I decided that the best thing for me would be to end my work with Claudia and move on. We had one more session in which we took time to review our journey together and say our good-byes.

What surprised me the most about this experience was how much self-understanding I gleaned from it *after* we had said good-bye. I did not begin working with a new Synergist for several weeks after our last session, and I used this interim to reflect on my process of closure with Claudia. In doing so, I gradually became aware of the origins of my fears about ending relationships and resolving conflict. What surfaced was a new understanding of an old behavior pattern: running away from conflict.

This behavior pattern had developed during my high school years, after a number of intense mentoring relationships had ended very abruptly and painfully. I was devastated by these losses and, with each one, told myself that I must have done something terrible; otherwise these wonderful people would not have hurt me as I felt they had. To avoid experiencing this kind of pain again, I had unwittingly adopted a pattern of emotionally abandoning a relationship the instant I perceived conflict or felt I had been wronged. I did not ask others to meet my needs for fear of being rejected outright, and, not wanting to experience again the devastation of being left, I was always prepared to leave first. In fact, most of my social relationships were quite peaceful, and I rarely felt forced to physically abandon anyone. Yet this was only due to my continued willingness to accept the hurt and pain of many relationships without speaking up for myself.

When I recognized the pattern, I saw how self-defeating it

was. Yet rejection by one party or the other was the only model of conflict resolution I'd had. When I began to feel uncomfortable with Claudia—no matter what the reason—it was only natural for me to feel like running away to protect myself. By creating a receptive and supportive environment in which I could discover my needs and fully express them, Claudia had helped me feel safe enough to stay and work through the fear of being left. Even as we were coming to closure, Claudia was providing me with a healthier model for resolving conflict, one that would support my ability to maintain meaningful relationships and, if need be, to say good-bye in a conscious way.

These insights into my old pattern of fleeing conflict did not flash on like a lightbulb, offering a new perspective, a new way of looking at things. My awareness of this pattern grew little by little, and I believe that I have been able to integrate it into my being all the more because of the gradual nature of the process. Like nutrients permeating the cells of my body, these insights seeped slowly and subtly into my conscious awareness. Eventually they became so fused with my core self that it was difficult for me to remember what it had been like to reflect on past relationships *without* my knowledge and understanding.

I know I can go back to Claudia any time I need to because neither one of us hurt, or was hurt by, the other. Neither one of us burned the bridge of our relationship, and in my contacts with her since our last session I have not felt ashamed or hurt, as I had in previous relationships. When I look back now at these past experiences within the framework of the closure process with Claudia, I see that it was my lack of conscious closure in the distant past that had fueled my anxiety over the prospect of leaving her.

I am now building upon the safety and completion I felt with Claudia throughout our process of closure, and I continue to integrate what I learned into my everyday life and relationships.

FROM INSIGHT TO
Integration

IT'S ONE THING to gain new insights about the origins of some of our unwanted behavior patterns. It's another to convert these insights into lasting changes in behavior. Getting from one to the other requires exploring alternative behaviors in order to find some that are more life-enhancing.

Fledgling behaviors need to be practiced if they are to survive in the real world, outside of sessions. Muscles that learn to relax on the table need to learn to stay relaxed while sitting, standing, and moving around. More complex behaviors also need to be integrated into daily life. Some clients are able to achieve significant and lasting change in behavior after only one or two sessions. More often, however, the process of integration takes months or years of ongoing work. The following stories illustrate various degrees of successful integration.

Synopses

I Can Take It! In a session, Jeanne has a visceral experience of the toll that her workaholism takes on her body. In another session two divergent characters in her imagined Greek drama provide Jeanne with images and awareness she can use outside of sessions for transforming her approach to work and life.

Letting Go of Grief. In two sessions with Gail, Fred* experiences long-overdue grief over the loss of his childhood pets and other family losses. Seven years after the second session, Fred writes to Gail about the major changes he has made since then in his life and relationships.

Self-Integration, Piece by Piece. Rob describes five key sessions—highlights from a five-year period during which he integrated many aspects of his physical and emotional awareness.

Breaking the Cycle of Pain-Fear-Pain. Peggy describes ten sessions with Ken,* who is depressed over having lost his job due to circulatory problems. Ken discovers that a habitual tension in his foot has been exacerbating the pain. When he learns to ease the tension, his self-esteem and mobility improve.

Life after Death. Patricia describes four memorable sessions that were milestones in her gradual recovery from feelings of guilt and loss over her son's suicide.

I Can Take It!

Jeanne Reock

"*Pile it on.* I can take it."

"More?"

"Yes, it's okay."

"More?"

"I can handle it."

And so it went as Joe Weldon, my Rubenfeld Synergist, placed more and more books on my body as I lay face up on a padded table. With my permission Joe was creating a physical experience that mirrored my inner experience, my sense that I can handle the heavy stuff.

The weight of the books had a certain sweetness about it at first. I felt a sense of pride in my ability to withstand the pressure. But eventually it grew heavy and oppressive. As my breathing became more and more difficult, I became acutely aware of the force deep inside me that drives me to take on more and more. It's a familiar force. It will not let me surrender. It holds me tough and lets me carry heavy burdens. Carrying the heavy stuff is what I'm supposed to do. That's what my life's about. That's what gives meaning to my days, weeks, and months.

I finally yielded to Joe's offer to remove some of the books. As he lifted them from my chest, I reveled in my newfound freedom to breathe easily. I moved and squirmed for the sheer joy of being able to. Every cell in my body rejoiced. A realization flooded me: I can stop at a comfortable point...or I can keep going until it really hurts—and beyond. It's my choice. It's all my choice, both in this small experiment and in my life. The choices I made during this experiment were a perfect metaphor for how I choose to live my life.

But which part of me does the choosing? While Joe stacked more and more books on top of me, the "I" who dominated my consciousness was the plucky, determined doer. This Determined One sees herself as strong, committed, and capable. She is known for her perseverance. I've been aware that she is a big part of me, often in control, with the consequence that I live much of my life feeling overburdened, having too much to do. Time becomes a scarce commodity, which must be used wisely and well because it is so precious. Every moment is a battleground: Whatever I'm doing, I feel I should be doing something else, which might accomplish more or be more important.

Then there is the other part of me, the Fair Witness. She observes and notices that I *do* place limits on my commitments. I have to. There are thousands, millions of things I could be doing and it's obvious that I can't do them all. So the Fair Witness wonders why I don't draw my boundaries at a more comfortable place.

None of these awarenesses were new to me in a conscious,

thinking sense. I already knew I take on so much that I feel over-burdened much of the time. What I was getting from this session was a visceral knowing. I literally felt my breath being cut off as the weight on me reached the outer limits of my tolerance. It was a familiar feeling and in that moment I became aware of how often I forget to breathe when I am intensely involved in turning out a piece of work. Oh, I breathe, but in a very shallow way, just enough to keep me alive and moving. What I miss is the deep, sustaining breath that gives me energy and life and fullness.

Immobilized under the mountain of books, I knew in my gut that I too often sacrifice my bodily comfort to the demands of do-ing a task. I thought of how I stay at the computer long after my back informs me that it is aching and sciatic pain has set in. Or how I make just one more phone call even though my ear hurts from the pressure and I'm tired of talking and listening and think-ing. I let the weight of my commitment to whatever I'm doing overwhelm my need to take care of myself.

Looking back on the session I see that Joe was the externali-zation of my Fair Witness, the part of me that keeps checking in to see how I'm doing and reminds me that I have a choice at every moment. Joe made this clear by asking for my permission at the beginning of the experiment and at every stage along the way. He constantly checked with me to see how I was doing. He was also compassionate, caring about the discomfort I was experiencing. And finally, he was wise enough to set things up so that I could become fully aware of the Determined One's power over me.

The book-piling session, as I came to think of it, was a land-mark in the ongoing work that I have been doing with Joe around this issue of feeling overburdened. I saw with a new compassion how I disregard my body's clear and abundant signals. Seeing this made some difference in how I spent my days and how I felt, but my old patterns still had a strong hold.

Several months later I had another powerful session with Joe on this same theme. This session took place at a very busy and burdened time for me—just two weeks before a national conference for which I had major responsibility. My head was spinning with all I had to do and with the anticipation of what was to come.

This time, as I was lying on the table with Joe's gentle hands cradling my head, an image came to me of a woman on a stage, a kind of classical Greek theater. With long hair and a flowing, ankle-length gown, she was a dramatic figure. I knew instantly that this Dramatic One was me—ranting and raving about all that I had to do, even beating my breast and shouting "Poor me!" or some guttural Greek version of that feeling.

To my surprise Joe asked who was on the stage with her. I replied without hesitation: the Wise Woman. She was a very attractive older woman, gray hair pulled back in a soft bun, dressed in a long skirt and boots and radiating a steady, strong, calm energy. Joe asked, "What does she say?"

I answered, "Calm down. It'll all get done. You've got time and you'll handle whatever comes up."

Joe suggested that I make room for her and disregard the Dramatic One's skepticism.

When Joe asked me what the Dramatic One sees when she looks out at the audience, I answered with amazement, "Nothing. It's just a black void." She's aware that there is an audience, but she doesn't really see them. They have no faces, no reality to her. She is totally alone in her drama.

The Wise Woman, however, sees the audience clearly and relates to each person there. She even sits on the edge of the stage and talks to them. She is interested in these people and cares about them, feeling connected to each of them, heart to heart. Their presence fills and pleases her.

The story that unfolded on the Greek stage in my mind was a

perfect metaphor for what happens in my life. Since these two sessions, and others that have deepened my learning on this theme, my life has been different. I now have images to call upon when I feel overburdened. I see myself more and more as the Wise Woman, confident that whatever is really important will get done in sufficient time without undue stress.

When the Dramatic One does show up nowadays, I ask her to leave the stage even before she starts ranting and raving. I just don't give her much space anymore.

As I make more room on my stage for the Wise Woman, my life is lighter. I take time to go sailing, sit in the sun, watch reruns of my favorite TV show, or chat with friends. What's even more important, I pay less attention to the chatter in my head that schedules and plans and worries about all the work I have yet to do.

Some days I am tempted to play the heavy, to be the overburdened workhorse. I feel the ache in my upper back and shoulders as I slip into the harness. Then I remember the Wise Woman and I see with her eyes that all my work is my choice, that it enriches my life in countless ways, and that it rarely needs to be done this very minute or even this very day. Some of it may actually never get done, and the world will continue to turn and the sun will rise tomorrow. That is so good to know.

Letting Go of Grief

Gail Benton

The first time I watched Ilana demonstrate the Rubenfeld Synergy Method, in 1987, I instantly recognized the mind–body connection from my own background in bodywork and psychotherapy. I had practiced for many years as a psychotherapist and had studied family systems, Ericksonian Hypnotherapy, and psychodrama. After having worked in a private agency as a social work clinician, I now owned and managed my own psychotherapy clinic and private practice.

I had also been a devoted yoga student and teacher for many years. With yoga I experienced the power of an integrating force between body and mind and a calming effect on the emotions. I went on to study massage, had many personal sessions of bodywork, and studied the body's subtleties of movement, sound, and breath. Yet I felt something was missing. When students' emotions emerged during classes, as sometimes happened, many of my yoga teachers either ignored these displays or downplayed their significance. The practitioners I saw for bodywork seemed to ignore it when I had an emotional reaction. And my psychotherapist colleagues seemed to dismiss the importance of the body, too, not understanding its "language" or the yoga concept of *chakras* (energy systems).

I wanted to integrate the changes that were happening in my body and in my life by incorporating my personal growth into my psychotherapy practice. Until I met Ilana, I had no way to do this on my own.

At that first workshop with Ilana, her demonstrations with "clients" selected from among the participants convinced me that I was on the right path—that it was safe for emotions to be experienced, understood, and integrated in the "here and now." At last I had a model for weaving together verbal therapy and bodywork. Now I would be able to effect more profound change than I could achieve with either approach alone.

Most important, during the first residential workshop with Ilana I was a "client" for her demonstration session in front of the group. This was the spark that ignited my interest in Rubenfeld Synergy. I remember working on the issue of making personal contact with others and creating my own personal boundaries. This was the beginning of a recurring theme in my life. In response to Ilana's respectful contact with me, my body began to change. I noticed that I carried my shoulders in a different way. I also felt that my heart and spirit had been freed in the process.

This was the first of many experiences in which I observed the power of this work. My personal and professional life would never be the same. Since then, through many experiences with Rubenfeld Synergy, all the major areas of my life have been touched and changed. I have experienced moments of ecstatic bliss, laughter, pathos, deep grief, and yearning. I feel that my soul has been cleansed and my body has become lighter and softer. I know that my energy flows more freely through me now, and I don't use so much of it to "contain" myself by stifling my impulses. I have greater freedom of movement. For me Rubenfeld Synergy is a process of becoming—a flow between body, mind, and spirit that takes a unique path every time.

In the six years since my training and certification in the Rubenfeld Synergy Method, I have grown increasingly interested in the results clients sometimes achieve with only a few sessions. I discovered this phenomenon inadvertently, when some of my clients were limited, by their managed care insurance, to "short-term therapy." I began to notice—to my surprise—that some clients reported dramatic changes that had occurred quickly and without any overt discussion or understanding of how or why they took place.

Fred,* a client I saw only twice, seven years ago, illustrates the kind of fast yet lasting change that Rubenfeld Synergy can foster. Sixty years old, Fred was on several medications for depression, back pain, arthritis, gastritis, and heart problems. He had difficulty motivating himself and did not feel like going to work. He had been impotent for about four years and was very frustrated by not having a more satisfying sexual relationship with his wife.

Although I did not use touch in my first session with Fred, Gestalt techniques helped him gradually increase his focus on his feelings as well as on his physical and emotional issues. We explored his grief over his father's death and the loss of his child-hood pets, from whom he had felt unconditional love. He became tearful as he described how he had never fully grieved over these losses or his failing health. He had not dealt with his son's drug problems or his daughter's divorce and remarriage. His mother, chronically depressed and anxious, was living in a nursing home. He began to recognize a pattern in how he dealt with unpleasant people or situations—by avoidance and withdrawal.

His first dog died when Fred was around three or four years old. He remembers squeezing and hugging another dog so much that he was crushing the dog's insides; his parents had to give the dog away, because he was harming it. The last dog was a golden retriever with whom he had a special relationship. He and the dog walked together every morning and Fred always felt total love and acceptance from him. In our session, at my urging, Fred spoke to each dog directly. He expressed the ways he appreciated and loved them, and he said good-bye to them. Fred also played the role of his dogs, giving Fred messages of love, acceptance, and approval. I guided Fred in integrating some of these affirmations for himself and gave him the suggestion that he could continue his walks—with or without his dogs—and take care of himself and his body. By the end of the session, Fred experienced some relief from pain and was breathing more easily. I gave him the "homework assignment" of noticing some of his appreciations every day.

At the start of our second session, Fred reported that something had opened up inside of him—especially with respect to grieving the loss of his dogs. He had begun communicating more with his wife and was feeling less depressed, even though the stresses in his life remained the same. He expressed concern that his oldest son had turned away from his faith.

In this session, as I used gentle touch Fred became aware that parts of his body were giving him messages to slow down, to pay attention, and to take better care of himself. He also got in touch more deeply with his grief over his father's death and his guilt that he had not made contact with his mother on the recent anniversary of his father's death. He was able to express how much he missed his father, how much he loved him, and how he could continue communicating with him in spirit form. As I supported his shoulders through touch, I gave him the suggestion that he could connect with his father without having to mimic the same aches and pains his father had suffered in his last years. Fred saw the connection between his father's expectations of him as a firstborn child and his own expectations of Ross,* his eldest (firstborn) son. I guided him in an imaginary conversation with Ross. Fred told Ross that he loved him despite Ross's having chosen a different path. Fred expressed his desire to communicate his love and care to Ross, and to tell him that he prays for him daily.

As I supported Fred's hips with my hands, we "reframed" his hip pain by looking at it from another point of view. Fred came to see the pain as an ally that would remind him when he ignored his body or overloaded himself with stress. I encouraged him to give himself and his body parts loving messages and reassurances that they could let go and not work so hard. His body shook visibly as he released what seemed to me to be blocked energy.

By the end of this session, Fred reported feeling very tall. His shoulders and chest were noticeably more open and relaxed, his face and eyes bright, and most of his muscles and joints more relaxed. He was hopeful that his life and relationship with his wife would continue to improve. Fred was able to see how he is connected to the universe and how God lives within him and also in the stars, the heavens, and the Earth. (He had been watching the Joseph Campbell television series, *The Power of Myth*.)

Fred did not schedule another session right away because he wanted to continue to integrate his new learnings and changes. He said he would return if his sexual intimacy problems persisted.

I didn't hear from Fred for seven years. When I phoned him recently in order to get permission to write about his sessions, he told me he had recently spent time with a longtime friend who was dying. Fred saw that, through having dealt with grief in his own life, he was able to help others. He followed up with a letter that brought me up to date on what has happened since completing our work together:

> *I can deal with grief better. I still have mood swings, and it's possible for me to get down on myself because of the depression. But I can talk about it and not be ashamed....Maybe that will help others deal with their own.... With regard to our sessions, you know when you hit on the idea of me talking to all my dogs one at a time, I was going back to around 1932. (I'm sure of the date because I wasn't in kindergarten yet.) That was an unexpected linkage between dogs/death/ grief and separation. I would put so much of myself into a dog that when they would run away I would feel as if they were rejecting me. Rejection—there's another one. I may not have been able to separate death from rejection.*
>
> *I was actually happy when my mother died because she no longer was the person I remembered and loved....I remembered that I hadn't kissed her good-bye or told her that I loved her so I went back and did that...and the next day the sheriff told us Mom was dead....It was a good time, as was the period around the funeral with my family.*

My brief work with Fred and others shows that profound and miraculous changes can and do occur when we honor all aspects of ourselves, reweave the past with the present, and release the blocked energy in our bodies, minds, and spirits.

Self-Integration

PIECE BY PIECE

Diane Junglas

The title of my doctoral dissertation was *The Experience of Becoming an Integrated Self Through Rubenfeld Synergy*. This topic does not lend itself to quantitative, double-blind studies. Instead I used a qualitative research method called heuristics, which includes the researcher's passion for and connection to the experience being studied.

The heuristics process investigates human experience by giving both the scientist and the participants (called co-researchers) the responsibility to be self-disclosing and rigorous in the pursuit of discovery and truth. One of my co-researchers was Rob Bauer. In five hours of in-depth, open-ended interviews in May 1993, Rob shared with me his subjective experience of becoming integrated through Rubenfeld Synergy.

Except for comments [shown in brackets], all of the following material comes from Rob's side of our interviews.

October 1988: Am I Acceptable?

I had completed my master's degree in social work and was starting to work as a psychotherapist. I realized something was missing. I was bored and wanted more than just sitting across from somebody, listening and talking. I went to a weekend workshop that Ilana was giving, and in the first ten minutes of being there I had an aha! experience:

> *This is what I want to be doing in my life.[1] This is the missing piece. The integration of body and mind in her work really feels right to me....I'm aware that my heart center[2] is a little more open. That's where I'm feeling it, in my heart center.*

I volunteered to do a demonstration session with Ilana in that workshop. The theme of my session was, basically, "Am I acceptable?" Ilana was able to elicit from me my "in-the-moment" experience—"You're a very nice lady and you're very pleasant and you're going to be very nice to me, but you will never accept me into your program 'cause you won't think that I am ready or evolved enough or intelligent enough or whatever." So that was what the session was about and by the end of it, Ilana had helped me feel empowered enough to ask for what I wanted.

That was my first of many sessions in my journey to integration over a five-year period. In that first session I took the message "I am acceptable" into my heart and mind, but not into my body. I don't remember being aware of my body or even of Ilana's touch during that session.

---

[1] Italics are used when Rob speaks about the sessions in the present tense.—*Ed.*

[2] Chest area. Same as *heart chakra*, seat of the emotions in Eastern systems.

July 1989: Pinocchio

I was in the training program and, halfway through the first year, I did my first demo with Ilana in front of the training group. In this session, through Ilana's use of touch, I began to feel my body in a new way. Of course I was already primed for this after half a year in the training group, with all the BodyMind Exercises about awareness, and touching and being touched in the small groups. I had begun to get some sense of my body and how rigid it was, how I held on to it and breathed shallowly.

As Ilana does the hip releases she asks me for an image about what I'm feeling in my legs, and I tell her how my legs feel like wood; both sides feel like wood. To explore this Ilana asks me about the color of the wood, the density of the wood, the kind of wood, more and more getting in touch with what it is like to feel wood. And I think she even says that wood is alive. It comes from a tree. Wood has energy in it; it is not a dead thing.

As she works with me, sometimes Ilana talks to the group about what's going on, and why she's doing what she's doing, and about what she's feeling.... Ilana tells the group, "This is so interesting. This man is lying here and talking about how dead he feels...in his legs, and I, Ilana, am feeling all this tremendous energy. So what's going on that he's not aware of it?" And, of course, I'm taking this in. On some level she's planting seeds and I'm ingesting that, and on some level I'm looking at that and saying, "Well, she's feeling energy!" I see that she is very subtly suggesting a different way for me to start to experience myself.

Ilana said, "Ohhh, it sounds like Pinocchio!" That was key. I burst out laughing, which Ilana immediately commented on.

·"Pinocchio" worked for me. Pinocchio had been a major figure in my childhood. When I was five or six years old and the
movie first came out, I went to see it at a drive-in in New Jersey
with my parents. It was a very scary movie, with the whale and the
cat and those evil types that kidnapped Pinocchio.

*And this little boy on his journey is seeing the dark side and
how scary all of that is. And all the time, I'm feeling more
and more in my legs. They're still wood, but they have feeling and I'm feeling the texture of them. One is smoother; one
is rougher. They are different colors.*

Then I came to statements that were so important to me. I said,
"I no longer want to sit on the shelf. And I don't want to have my
strings pulled. And I don't want to be manipulated." Those were
awarenesses that came out of being Pinocchio, being a mari-
onette. Of course, later on, when it came time to choose the title
of the piece,[3] I named it *Pinocchio.*

The final part of the *Pinocchio* piece was getting off the table
and feeling myself on the floor, having these wooden legs that
now had life in them, sensing that wood could breathe, wood
could be alive, and feeling what it was like to walk with these
wooden legs that were not so wooden anymore. There was some
flexibility in this wood, some breath that went through it....I was
feeling the contact of the floor underneath me, feeling the carpet
through the soles of my feet. I was extremely conscious of the texture of the carpet, almost feeling each fiber in the carpet tickling
or making contact with me—sending energy to me, just as I had
felt energy from Ilana's touch....As I walked around, I came to
the undercarpet, where the Oriental rug left off. Placing one foot

---

[3] After each demonstration session, the client is asked to name the session or "piece of personal work."

on each carpet, I appreciated the difference coming through each foot. It reminded me of being at the seashore with one foot in the water and one in the sand. I was really tranced out in this extraordinary deep place of feeling the carpets.…This experience is still with me after five years. I still have that awareness in my body.

February 1990: I Am the Gong

In my second year of training, I had a session with Ilana at a film studio because it was to be used in a documentary. We started the session with Ilana asking me about my job. I had a part-time therapy practice on my one day off, but my main job was working in a theater box office—fifty or sixty hours a week in the busy season. It was all work; I had no time to just live.

Ilana asked where in my life I would like to be. I recalled a major experience in my life—being at Omega [Omega Institute for Holistic Studies, a learning community in Rhinebeck, New York]. This was in the late seventies, when Omega was in its infancy, with only about fifty students and a few teachers. We were a small group that had the chance to bond and be very intimate. Everybody volunteered to do things. I volunteered to be the dishwasher and I loved it because it was my idea. I would chuckle, "If my friends in New York and all those theater people could only see me now!" I was in my element.

Omega was the beginning of a major process for me because, that very first summer, I did a meditation course. That was the first time anyone told me that I didn't breathe properly, and the first time I became aware of how much pain I had in my back, especially in my left shoulder—my "left wing"—the heart center of the back. Omega was perhaps the first place that I felt totally accepted. People kept encouraging me to move into the holistic field. I was studying nutrition and Polarity Therapy and herbs.

At Omega I had so much energy that I woke up at five in the morning. That was quite extraordinary, because in New York City I couldn't even get up when the alarm went off, and I'd have to drag myself to wherever I was going. Yet here at Omega, I had all this energy. I was up with the birds, up with the sunrise. I was the first one up and I'd walk on the lawn in my bare feet and feel the dew on my feet and feel free. There was a big bell on the lawn at Omega, and I began ringing the bell. I became the bell ringer, awakening everybody at the dawn of the new day. I loved it!

As I talk about that summer Ilana senses in my body the joy of ringing the bell, so she encourages me to ring it. Lying on the table I swing my right arm—dong, dong, dong—back and forth, just allowing more of my body to get into the act of ringing the bell, swinging my arm and my shoulder, ring-ing in the new day, new beginnings.

I started opening up in my chest and breathing more deeply. I said, "I am free here under the sky. I can just ring the new begin-ning of my life." I began to integrate the message that I can become free *of* my life and free *in* my life.

January 1991: Wild Horse of Living

In the final year of my training, I did another demo with Ilana in front of the training group. Although I had not yet graduated, I was already on the staff of the next training class. That was major for me, being invited to be on staff. I didn't have time to get into my scary place and say, "Do you mean it?" I had to just get out there and do it, whether or not I felt I could do it. And then I found I could! Exhausting as the staffwork was, it forced quantum leaps in my growth. I moved into really taking the reins of power, which, it turned out, was what this session was about.

At the time, I was very fearful about a friend who was having a health crisis. Ilana helped me realize that my fear had to do with my mother, who had abandoned me by dying when I was thirteen, and my father, who died soon after that. Whenever people got sick I would become afraid that they would die and leave me, too. I felt it wasn't safe to get too close to them. Ilana helped me understand that I was projecting onto my friend my feelings of abandonment by my mother. She helped me see that I didn't have to be responsible for my friend. I could help him without being responsible for him. I realized then that when I was a teenager I had felt responsible for my parents during their final illnesses.

This *Wild Horse of Living* session was about taking my reins of power—knowing that I could gallop free on the plain and not have to take care of everybody else. I could be me and fly with the wind like a horse wherever I wanted to go—be the stallion, be the steed, be free and really feel the power in my body. In that session I got more and more in touch with the integration of my whole body, not just like in the *Pinocchio*, in the bottom half, or in *I Am the Gong*, somewhat of the top half. Now my whole body could gallop across the plain and go where it wanted to go—and not even know where it was going—and that was okay.

The following day I made the commitment to leave my box office job as soon as the theater season was over, and to start a full-time practice.

August 1992: Eagle's Wing

Last summer a group of us went to Orcas Island to spend a week with Werner [Kundig]. We each got to do a session with Werner as part of the package. I began my session by chatting with him. I joked that the real reason I was there was because he had said eagles flew near the house. I was really drawn to the eagle and wanted to embrace it as my power symbol, and that was what brought me there—not Werner.

He and I worked on what that was all about, this eagle that I wanted to be. We got in touch with the pain that I have had in my left shoulder ever since an accident years ago. I had injured the sixth cervical vertebra and had pain in my upper back, basically around the heart *chakra* on the back. The pain was also related to my need to open the heart center. When I hold emotional tension there, it manifests as back pain.

Werner's bodywork really got into that pain and evoked a lot of sadness and deep feelings about how I, the eagle, do not fly. I have one good wing and one injured wing, and I can't fly well with an injured wing. So I sit in the nest and don't fly free. This session was the next step toward being able to fly in the air, not just gallop on the plain. We worked to discover what keeps me in the nest. We followed a metaphor of my flying with the injured wing. Then I saw myself as an eagle flying out and falling into the sea, going right down to the bottom and not resurfacing—staying down underneath the water with my broken wing. And I got in touch with the fear.

It was important for me to recognize that I wanted to reclaim my wing, mend my wing, empower myself and fly. By the end of the session I wasn't there yet, but I recognized that I had a major fear of flying.

May 1993

I had two private sessions with Werner during a training week in New York. We started by reviewing what had happened during the previous training week, in February, when my upper back had gone into spasm. The pain was so bad that I had spent the whole week lying flat on my back. We talked about the stress and strain

I experience when I play the caretaker role—feeling that it is not okay for me to set boundaries by saying, "No, I can't give you that."

This discussion led into another exploration of allowing myself to be me—allowing myself to be exhausted, to say no, to say yes—so that when I say yes, it will really come from choosing to say yes. I discovered I had a lot of confusion about that, so it was hard for me to be present when I wanted to say yes.

After these sessions I noticed that I felt different in my body and that my soul felt so much better. I was powerful in a different way. I needed less to be in control, I could trust [fellow staff members] more. I began to supervise trainees differently, too. I was present and focused with the them and supported them from my own position, without having to be off-balance from caretaking them. I saw that they could feel empowered just from my being present with them.

THESE SESSIONS with Ilana and Werner were milestones in my process of integration—getting to own every part of myself. In the first session, *Am I Acceptable?*, I was closed off, peeking through a crack in the door and asking, "Am I really okay? Can I trust you?" I was not aware of my body or Ilana's touch in that session. In *Pinocchio* I started to experience my body, especially the hips and legs. I began to walk on and feel the ground underneath me, instead of tiptoeing around. In *I Am the Gong* I began to incorporate the upper half of my body. Swinging my arms and my shoulders, I began to open my chest and breathe more deeply, and to see the possibility of real change in my life. In *Wild Horse of Living* I got in touch with my whole body and began to take the reins of power in my life—literally and figuratively. In *Eagle's Wing* I recognized my fear of allowing my life to "take off" and my commitment to healing my broken wing. The private sessions dealt with extending my own healing to others by just being.

Integration is a gradual process. First there is a heightened awareness; then comes movement toward empowerment. In my case something that had started as a cognitive awareness then moved into my psyche, where it opened up my heart and soul a little before beginning to penetrate into my body, going all the way down. Looking back, it's easy to see the progression.

Breaking the Cycle of Pain-Fear-Pain

Peggy Kostyshyn

When I first saw Ken a year ago, he had just received bad news from the cardiovascular surgeons. They told him that the last of five surgeries to restore circulation to his right leg had failed and that he should "just go home and learn to live with it." So much scar tissue had developed from the surgeries that another incision might not be able to heal. And if his condition worsened, they might need to amputate his leg.

Despite his daily regimen of painkillers, Ken could not walk far before the pain forced him to stop. He had been forced out of his supervisory job because of his disability, and was living on an early-retirement pension. Although he was depressed, Ken was not a quitter. At fifty-two he felt he was too young to give up on himself without a good fight. He had never been particularly interested in health issues, nor had he any experience with any kind of therapy, psychological or physical. Desperate to escape disability, though, he started to look into the body–mind connection. That's when he called me to inquire about Rubenfeld Synergy.

I have seen Ken twenty times over the last year. In the first four sessions, last fall, he dealt mainly with his fears, his hopes, and the essence of who he is—with or without his right leg. Then in six sessions last spring, he became aware of many holding patterns in his body, especially how his left hip and leg had taken over most of the work of his right hip and leg. And now, this summer, we have worked together twice a week for the last five weeks. I am astonished by the breakthroughs Ken has made—not only in his outlook on life but also regarding his recovery from pain and his increased functioning in daily living. Here are synopses of this summer's sessions.

SESSION 1: Ken told me that he was getting a painful callus on the bottom of his right foot, over the fourth metatarsal head. I watched him walk around and asked him to notice how he was bearing weight on his feet. Then I had him soften his knees and notice what it felt like when he bore more weight on his heels and up through his spine. When he resumed his initial stance, bearing most of the weight on his toes, he was surprised that he felt immediately anxious.

SESSION 2: Ken said he was walking differently and that his wife had noticed it, too.

SESSIONS 3 THROUGH 5: We dealt with Ken's need to be busy and productive in order for him to feel that he has value. We touched on family themes, breathing, body awareness, and holding patterns.

SESSION 6: Wringing his hands as if twisting a towel, Ken demonstrated to me how his whole lower right leg and foot felt like a tightly twisted elastic. When he was lying on the table I noticed that both feet were pointed, with the toes curled under. Examining his feet more closely I noticed that on the sole of his right foot, the tendon connecting his heel to his great toe was tight and contracted. He was initially unaware of this tension even when I ran my fingers over the tendon and asked what he was aware of in that area. By session's end he was quite aware of it and also of the tightness in his Achilles tendon and hamstrings.

SESSION 7: As I had noticed in several previous sessions, Ken's right foot was so contracted at the beginning of the session that it appeared smaller than his left foot. With Ken sitting on the table and his feet resting on a stool, I gently encouraged the bones of each foot to spread by pressing in a certain way on the sole. Ken watched with interest as both feet relaxed and broadened, his right foot becoming as broad and full as his left.

SESSION 8: Ken arrived complaining about soreness in his right great toe. I asked him to remove his sock and sit on the table as I examined his foot. The great toe was curled up and over, toward the second toe, almost overlapping it. The large tendon on the top of his foot, which connects the great toe to the ankle, was so tight that even Ken could see it. Cradling his foot with both my hands I asked him what the foot and toe were trying to tell him.

Ken looked at me, puzzled. Then his face lit up and he said, "It's fear. I'm so afraid of injuring my toe—and getting gangrene and needing an amputation—that I curl it up to protect it. The pain's not from lack of circulation; it's a muscle spasm." He was intrigued by this awareness. "No wonder I have a callus on my foot!" he added. "I'm not walking properly."

SESSION 9: Three days later Ken announced with great pride that he was walking differently and using his great toe. He had no pain in the toe, foot, or leg. "It was all fear! And my right foot has stayed as wide as the left one since I left here Monday."

SESSION 10: This session focused on Ken's plans to travel to some of the places he had never taken time to see. He has found a rich reward in his forced early retirement—finding himself and enjoying life, feeling "like an adolescent for the first time." Ken credits these changes—his new lease on life and his new belief in himself—to the Rubenfeld Synergy process.

On a more mundane level, Ken said he "checks in" on his feet frequently. Sometimes he finds the toes of both feet relaxed and spread out. Sometimes he notices that his great toe has reverted to its old protective habit. When that happens he simply lets it relax to a more normal position. The callus on his foot is softening and disappearing. He feels he won't need the orthotic insert that was prescribed for him only three weeks earlier.

Ken has resumed hobbies and safe sports like bike riding. Although he won't ever be able to work full-time due to his blocked arteries, Ken wants to be productive and has begun to look into volunteer work.

He is a real believer in the Rubenfeld Synergy Method and in his own ability to affect his health. Although he acknowledges my guidance and teaching, he often tells me that he knows he has healed himself. And I agree.

Life after Death

Patricia Ellen

Seven months after the death of my fourteen-year-old son I was still falling apart, shattered and deeply remorseful. A planned trip fell through at the last minute, when I most needed to get away. Terrified of so much unstructured time, I began frantically to go through catalogs of retreat centers to find a replacement activity for that weekend.

As coincidence (or my guardian angels) would have it, I found a weekend workshop titled "Integrating Body, Mind, and Spirit," to be led by a woman named Ilana Rubenfeld. I'd never heard her name before, but integrating body, mind, and spirit seemed to promise just what I needed. And so, with a phone call, I registered and was off to experience the change of my life.

During the weekend Ilana kept telling us how Rubenfeld

Synergy could allow us to have more joy in our lives. Being the ever-compliant child, I tried and tried to feel joy but couldn't. Then I started to get angry. How could this woman expect me— a mother who had lost her child only seven months earlier—to have joy? I approached this Ilana person and told her exactly that. I didn't know it at the time, but I had just given her the perfect opening to invite me to be her "demo client." And when she did invite me up to experience a Rubenfeld Synergy session with her, I was stunned and shocked—and still obedient. I lay on the table and immediately relaxed into a light trance.

> Ilana touches my head and cradles it. There is something so safe about this touch that I begin to cry. Ever-so-gently Ilana leads me into the deep tears and rage that I have been feeling ever since Doug's death. She does not seem frightened as I reexperience the deepest pain I have ever known. As she moves from my head to my arms, then my feet, her gentle touch invites my tense muscles to let go. I sense her calmness, her total presence as a witness to whatever I might feel.
>
> Ilana asks me to put words to what I am feeling. I talk about my guilt and my sense of failure as a mother. I cry and cry. Gently, slowly, Ilana helps me connect with my inner self. As I begin to listen to the timid, nurturing voice within me, instead of to the loud critical voice, Ilana continues to touch my shoulders and hold me gently. I begin to discover the self that remembers I am a good mother, the self that knows Doug's suicide wasn't all my responsibility, the self that knows I was only a part of the whole picture. At Ilana's suggestion I keep repeating two phrases: "I am a good mother" and "I am only part of the whole picture." These phrases are like salve to a savage wound.

After I sit up Ilana has me walk around the healing circle of workshop participants. I look people in the eye and repeat my key phrase, "I am a good mother and I am only part of the whole picture." With each encounter my burden of guilt and shame lessens some more.

Then Ilana says, "Go home and make signs for your refrigerator to remind you of what you know here today." (I did just that and today, ten years later, I still have the signs—the first signposts on my journey of healing.)

As the session closes I stand in a circle holding hands with all those present, feeling a connection, love, and compassion that help me know that in some way I will survive this tragedy. And I know that someday, too, I will again be able to feel joy.

Leaving for home that Sunday afternoon, I knew something profound had happened. I knew that that one session of Rubenfeld Synergy had created more healing than four months of psychotherapy. My soul knew I needed to receive more Rubenfeld Synergy sessions, to heal from my trauma by releasing it from my body. My heart wanted to do this work. But my head was resistant and skeptical: Why did I want to spend all this time and money? Still, I kept thinking about this miraculous method and, seven months later, I began the Rubenfeld Synergy Training Program and my journey to wholeness.

One of the training requirements was to have sessions with different Rubenfeld Synergists. What a gift that requirement was to my soul! One of these healers was Werner Kundig, who with touch and words could coax even the deepest muscles to relax. As we worked with images, I was able to release ever-deeper layers of feelings.

One session found me screaming in rage and sorrow at Doug.

"How could you have done this to me and to your sister! Why? Why? Why?" As I screamed and cried, Werner's touch guided the energy I was releasing up my spine and out of my body. With each subsequent session I released more and more of the trauma from my body. And with each release Werner's gentle touch was like a mother's kiss to make it all better.

After many such sessions Werner invited me to imagine that Doug was there with me. What did I have left to say to Doug? I told him how much I missed him, how much I appreciated all we had shared in his time on this Earth. I told him I didn't want to forget or lose him. As I talked with Doug, Werner encouraged me to find a place in my body where I felt I wanted to keep him. Instantly I knew I would place Doug in my heart and carry him with me wherever I went.

One Year Later: Releasing the Guilt

During each week of the training, Ilana did several demonstration sessions with trainees taking turns as "client." One week, nineteen months after Doug's death, I was feeling particularly dismal and depressed. She must have sensed it because she asked me to be the client. I jumped at the chance to work with her again.

> In the center of the healing circle, Ilana sits in one chair and invites me to sit in the other. Without touching me, she guides me with gentle questions. "What are you feeling in your body?"
>
> "A burden of guilt on my back," I respond. "It's stopping my life."
>
> Ilana asks for a third chair to be brought into the circle. She names this chair "Guilt" and invites me to move to this new chair, to play the role of Guilt—to see what Guilt wants to say to me. As Guilt I say to the chair representing

me, "Patricia, you are responsible for the loss of a life. You have no right to go on and be happy. You owe it to Doug to stay miserable. That is the least you can do to make it up to him."

Ilana asks me to move back to the chair representing Patricia. In this chair I can't think of anything to say to Guilt. Reluctantly I agree that I have no right to be happy. Ilana asks for a fourth chair, to represent Doug. She asks me to look at that chair and speak to Doug. I tell Doug, "I would have done anything to stop you, if only you had let me know how bad you felt."

Ilana asks me to sit in Doug's chair and speak as Doug. "Doug" responds to Patricia: "I didn't want to bother you. I didn't know it was this bad. I thought I could handle it on my own. I kept telling you everything was fine."

As we carry on this dialogue, it slowly dawns on me that these phrases sound familiar. "I don't want to bother you." "I think I can handle it on my own." "Everything is fine." These phrases express exactly what I do when I am feeling upset. I don't want to bother anyone. I can handle it by myself. This is what Doug had learned from my example, from his father's example, and maybe even from society. This is an aha! moment for me—a moment of clarity—albeit a very painful one.

With this realization my focus switches to myself and how I deal with painful feelings. I begin to see my "pressure cooker" pattern of releasing pain. Because I don't want to bother anyone with my scary feelings, and because I am terrified that these feelings will overwhelm me and destroy me, I let them escape a little at a time. I keep the lid on and try to handle my feelings on my own, all the while telling everyone—and myself—that everything is fine.

I also realize that greater than my fear of the feelings themselves is my fear of having someone see my feelings, of having someone see me as ugly and repulsive for having these feelings, of having someone reject me because I don't look happy. So I keep my pain to myself. I am left with letting off steam, just a little at a time, so it won't kill me as I handle it all alone.

All of these awarenesses pour through me in just a few moments. I begin to say them aloud to Ilana. I tell her, "I do want to do it differently. I do want to learn to risk sharing my pain. I don't want to go and hide as Doug did. I want to learn to feel my feelings when I am with people."

At that moment Ilana places her hands gently on my back and chest. I feel her touch as support. It is the first time she's touched me this entire session. Physically I am no longer alone. My body gets to experience that I am no longer doing this all alone. Ilana has me practice my new intention right away by encouraging me to invite an ally, someone to help me with my pain. I ask my classmate Jamie to come up to help me.

As the session proceeds I describe to Jamie and Ilana the gray mush that seems to surround me and keep me separate from other people. "The gray mush is very clever," I tell them. "I can let people think they are seeing me; I can get some contact but I remain protected and separate." The difficulty is that the gray mush of guilt is keeping me from having a life. I feel the gray mush overpowering me. I begin to wonder if maybe this was how Doug felt. I consider that this may have been how he was overpowered by his despair.

I decide I want to be rid of the gray mush and not be overpowered by it any longer. Ilana remarks that, during the session, she has observed me speaking and blowing out air with deep sighs. At her suggestion I exaggerate this blowing out over and over. As I do so I realize I am trying to blow that gray mush away. I want to be free to have contact with others.

Powerful play ensues. I ask Jamie to help me blow the gray mush away. Jamie agrees and takes my hand. Again my body experiences that I am not alone. Jamie and I begin to blow the gray mush away. Over and over we purse our lips, blow at the mush, and laugh. Soon we are playing like two children. When we feel that blowing is not getting rid of the gray mush fast enough, we create a fire hose to hose it down and wash the gray mush away. Finally we create great buckets of water to slosh it away. Slosh! Slosh! Slosh! As the gray mush disappears, I feel lighter and lighter. I feel young and free and playful. What a delight!

As the session comes to an end I find myself saying to Ilana, "This feels so easy. It feels strange and wonderful. It didn't hurt." I realize that when waves of guilt and gray mush engulf me, I can call someone and play them away. As this realization sinks in, Ilana reminds me that this is a different way of doing it, different from the way I've always done it, different from the way Doug did it. I feel I'm beginning to heal a very old and deep pattern. I am amazed that this healing has begun—without agony!—with ease, gentleness, and laughter. I didn't have to tough it out alone.

I returned home with new awareness: Healing doesn't have to hurt; there is life after guilt; I don't have to give up my life as Doug did; I don't have to tough it out alone; my mind and body can experience new ways of being and allow more contact with others.

Another Year Later: Juicy for Life

Three training weeks later (or one year later, depending on how you count), after having had some twenty sessions with different Rubenfeld Synergists, I volunteered to be Ilana's demonstration client. Volunteering was a major shift for me. The previous times, I had been in such pain that she'd had to ask me to be the client. This time I reached out and asked her to work with me. Reaching out was what the gray mush session had been all about.

So eager am I to have this session that I "claim" the demo table by placing my necklace on it. I want this session to celebrate how good I've been feeling. I tell Ilana that I am loving my work and enjoying my life—that I'm even in love. I also tell her about my recent attempts at home to imagine a Rubenfeld Synergy session with her, Ilana, as the Synergist. Unable to finish these imaginary sessions, I've decided to try the real thing.

Ilana smiles and asks me to describe these sessions. I tell her they focus on the split I've noticed recently between my warm hands and my cold feet. I explain that after Doug's death, I often noticed that my hands were suddenly warm. I would feel them pulsate with a kind of energy that was hard to describe, even to myself, because I had never felt anything like it before. I had quickly interpreted this warmth as a gift of healing energy that I was receiving from Doug. It was this new energy in my hands that had drawn me to Rubenfeld Synergy—as a vehicle for using the energy in healing others. Now I am concerned about the lack of warmth in my feet.

I tell Ilana, "The contrast between my warm hands and

cold feet came up in my last session and I want to heal this split."

Ilana asks me, "What do you think I would do as Synergist?" In her subtle way she is affirming that I have all the knowledge I need to find the answer on my own.

After struggling for an answer I finally say, "You would help me find a way to connect my hands and my feet."

The session continues with Ilana suggesting, "Let's have your hands and feet talk to each other."

My hands begin the conversation, saying to the feet, "We don't need you. You are extraneous."

Immediately my feet retort, "If you leave us out, you are going to fall over, Babe."

My hands are mute. They don't know how to respond.

All the while, as I lie on my back, Ilana is performing classic Rubenfeld Synergy moves to encourage the muscles of my arms and legs to relax and release their holding patterns. In the process she has bent and raised my knees so that they point to the ceiling and the soles of my feet are grounded on the table.

Once again seated at my head, Ilana asks what my hands have to say. I am still blank, my hands still mute. Ilana suggests that I let my hands speak for themselves and have a consultation with each other. She takes my hands in hers and moves them back and forth like two puppets conferring and giggling with each other. Laughter ensues, which gets me past my block and lets me go deeper inside.

I become aware of a shift in my energy—now my hands are feeling very cool. I say, "My hands have nothing to say. They are cold and they are scared. They don't know how to respond to the feet." With a great sense of uneasiness I say to Ilana, "I thought I had this all figured out...."

She reassures me that my work around Doug's death is not yet finished, that there is a piece still to be integrated. The calm, soothing quality of her voice invites me to relax. Still holding my hands Ilana says, "Let your hands finish this sentence. 'I'm scared of...'"

My hands keep gesturing as the responses come, slowly at first, then faster: "I'm scared of being foolish....I'm scared of letting go....I'm scared of losing Doug. I'm scared of losing energy in my hands and losing contact with Doug."

Bingo! We have hit the core of what is happening. Still holding my hands she asks me, "Sooooo, you are supposed to be sad forever?"

I nod and tell her that now, feeling wonderful and getting on with my life, I'm afraid I might lose my connection with Doug. As I say this I realize that my feet represent getting on with life. And cold feet are my fear that getting on will mean leaving Doug behind.

Ilana asks me to close my eyes. As I do so, suddenly I remember my necklace—the necklace I'd used to claim the table, the necklace Doug had given me! "Where is the necklace?" I ask. "In my pocket." Ilana pulls it out of her pocket and places it on my heart.

Instantly I feel my body relax. I am feeling very connected to Doug through my heart, the same heart connection I had experienced in my earlier work with Werner.

Ilana asks me to speak to Doug. I tell him I am happy, life is good, I love my work, and I have a new man in my life. "I no longer get sad every time I look at your picture. I don't want you to think I've forgotten you. I just don't want to be sad anymore."

Ilana reminds me that now I can be connected to Doug through my heart as well as my hands. As I lie there on the table, I am surrounded by an incredible sense of peacefulness in my heart, and of connection with Doug. Ilana's hands are still on my shoulders. She is silent for such a long time that I ask her if I should be doing something more. She assures me she is simply enjoying the peacefulness of the moment. I feel connected to Doug and to Ilana at the same time. Heaven and Earth.

I notice that my feet have started to warm up, and my hands as well. The peaceful pleasure spreads through my whole body. I realize that I am very much alive, alive with pleasure. Life feels juicy and I can connect with Doug in a whole new way—through my celebration of life.

As the Years Pass: "L'Chayim!"

Back home I started to experience more frequent moments of celebration. I began remembering, with joy, times I spent with Doug when he was a child. Present moments with my daughter, Lori, took on a precious quality. Sunsets became more intense. Stopping just to smell a flower or watch a butterfly became a sacred experience.

It has been ten years now since Doug shot himself and died. I know that the trauma will remain with me for the rest of my life. From time to time new layers of the old pain and trauma surface. Each time a new layer opens to be healed, I am able to use the tools of the Rubenfeld Synergy Method to experience the sadness or fear or rage, reach out to others for assistance, and move gently through the pain to peace and celebration of life.

Life after the death of a child is never the same. I have chosen transformation over living death and grief. Rubenfeld Synergy fostered that transformation through the hands, hearts, minds, and souls of many Synergists. My life journey continues drawing me ever closer to being fully alive—always with an awareness of the blessing of Doug's spirit, which I shared for fourteen years on this Earth and will share in my heart forever.

How We Learn
TO DO RUBENFELD SYNERGY

WHEN GIVING a session, a Rubenfeld Synergist needs to keep track of many things at the same time: the verbal "story" the client tells, often in a fragmentary way; how the client moves; changes in the client's breathing, voice quality, facial expression and complexion; everything the Synergist is doing and saying.

In Rubenfeld Synergy Training the requisite somatic and verbal skills are first taught separately. Their seamless coordination is learned through countless hours of demonstration, practice in small groups under supervision, and independent projects.

Many trainees are counselors, social workers, psychologists, or psychotherapists who want to go beyond the limitations of talk without touch. Many others are massage therapists, physicians, chiropractors, physical therapists, or other practitioners trained in the use of touch who want to learn how to support their clients' emotional responses. The rest are making a more dramatic break from careers outside the healing professions.

Synopses

The First Time Ilana Touched Me. Mike's process of unraveling his anger begins on the second day of his training, when Ilana touches his shoulder in passing.

My Body Suits Me Fine. During pauses in the daily Body-Mind Exercises in her first year of training, Barbara creates an exercise of her own that increases her awareness of her body's actual size and shape. This awareness gradually transforms her distorted body image, a remnant of a previous eating disorder.

Transforming Wounds into Possibilities. During Lee's demonstration session with Ilana in the first year of training, Lee contacts and releases feelings of guilt over her inability as a child to protect her younger sisters from sexual abuse.

What I Learned in the Pauses. Ilana demonstrates a new somatic technique to the class by having one of the trainees practice it on Meg, the demonstration client. Meg gains valuable insights as she lies quietly on the table.

Reflections. Annie recalls particular highlights of the training for which she crossed an ocean. She learns to trust her instincts and take risks.

Seasoned by Celeste. When Celeste* sits bolt upright during her first session as his nonpaying "practice client," Bill discovers that these practice sessions really *are* all about his own learning.

BodyMind Exercises. Peggy gains relief from symptoms of post traumatic stress disorder through her regular practice of Rubenfeld Synergy BodyMind Exercises.

I've Got To Be Travelin' On. Valerie is surprised that she has not totally recovered emotionally from her double mastectomy. She describes the process of integration that begins during her demonstration session with Ilana.

Intention. Instead of writing the required essay to explain what she learned about the intentions of Rubenfeld Synergy in her first year of training, Lee writes a poem.

The Eye of Memory. Lydia, who has videotaped over a hundred demonstration sessions during Rubenfeld Synergy trainings, shares her experience from behind the lens.

The First Time
Ilana Touched Me

Mike Schlesinger

The first time Ilana Rubenfeld touched me, I felt a rush of energy in my body unlike anything I had ever experienced. It was on the second day of my three-year training with her. I was not having a session with Ilana; I was sitting on the floor among other trainees and she just touched my left shoulder as she reached over me to adjust the air conditioner behind me. A rush of heat and energy came through my shoulder.

Ilana seemed to notice my reaction and that something powerful had happened because she put both of her hands on my right shoulder, rested them there for a few moments, then lightly slid them down my arm to my elbow and tossed them with a shrug into the air, as if to cast something off. Almost immediately an even greater flow of warmth and "aliveness" passed down from my shoulder and through my arm, and I felt a happy sense of well-being.

I had entered this training program after twenty years as a psychologist working mostly with severely ill psychiatric patients in state mental hospitals. Their diagnoses included paranoid schizophrenia, depression, bipolar (manic-depressive) disorders, antisocial personality disorders, and an assortment of organic brain syndromes. Despite spending so much time with people who were mentally ill, all in all my life was going pretty well, and I had a sense of stability and being rooted—not only in my work but also in my relationships. After twenty years I was still married to the same woman and I felt happy at home with her and our teenage kids—most of the time. Sometimes, however, I saw them as careless, selfish, or unappreciative, and then I would become either loud and angry or withdrawn and silent.

Through years of introspection, reading, and talking with my wife and friends—many of whom are also psychologists and therapists—I had come to understand that many of my interpretations and reactions had been passed down to me by my parents. They had lived through very hard times and had suffered a great deal. Since childhood they had been uprooted many times by the most horrendous, traumatic events—the First World War, the Great Depression, the Holocaust, and finally the Communist takeover of Eastern Europe. Growing up, I had heard their stories many times and some of their feelings of loss, fear, and rage had taken root inside of me as well.

So even though I loved my wife and kids and had learned that, for me, anger was often a cover for other feelings, especially fear and sadness, I still became critical and angry at times. I sensed that I often "held back" in my body and that I was restricted in my movements and energy. Furthermore, whenever I was sad I felt constricted in my throat and could not cry.

I understood how these energy blocks had formed: I clearly remembered my father's forbidding me to cry, and threatening that if I didn't stop the tears he would give me a real reason to cry. But understanding the source of these blocks had not released me from anger's grip. When I realized that my father's need to control was driven by his fear that I might get into trouble or be hurt, I forgave him, but even that did not release me from the anger.

Though I was content most of the time, I knew that my happiness and functioning—not to mention the happiness of those who lived with me—were limited by these unresolved issues of anger and control. I decided that I was ready to face my demons again, but this time I would deal with them at another level, through therapy that included bodywork as well as talk. I had been hearing about Ilana Rubenfeld's work since the midseventies, so when she gave a two-day workshop near my neighborhood I went to check it out.

I found her explanation of her background interesting, and I enjoyed the movement and awareness activities she led. I was impressed by her demonstration of the work, especially the way it created a therapeutic space of safety. I could imagine myself on her table, increasing my awareness of my body and myself, and, with her gentle verbal and physical support, possibly recalling traumatic events, reexperiencing them and resolving them. I also liked her energy, humor, and accepting attitude. Thinking that her approach might help me in my quest, I decided to apply for the three-year training program.

Even after I was accepted, and even after I arrived in New York, excited and curious, I still wasn't sure how much of myself I was ready to commit to learning and practicing Rubenfeld Synergy. But after I experienced Ilana's touch, I decided that I would volunteer to come up to the table for a session with her in front of the group. I was the first to raise my hand that afternoon. Ilana chose me and I spent the next forty-five minutes changing my life.

At the time it didn't seem like much. Ilana touched my head and feet as I lay on the table and we talked easily about my feet, my family, my life. Then, as she gently moved my legs and my arms and I gradually became more aware of my body, I noted some tension in my hips and shoulders. Ilana suggested that I carry on a dialogue with them. Soon she invited me to go back to a time when I had felt this tension more strongly. I told of sitting around the dinner table as a teenager and the tension I had felt then, when my parents nagged me about eating more, sitting up straight, not dawdling. While I talked Ilana performed her "magic" via releases of blocked energy—from my shoulders down through my arms, and from my hips down through my legs. And I noticed a lessening of the tension I carry in my chest, my throat, and my eyes. And that was all that happened in that session.

For the rest of that first week I watched Ilana demonstrate sessions with several of my classmates, and I saw them reveal their wounds and begin to heal. Some of these sessions included movement or music, and some used humor to bring light into the dark places. In addition to giving these daily demonstration sessions Ilana lectured and demonstrated "the listening touch" and some basic movements, which we then practiced in small groups under supervision. We also participated in body awareness classes based on the work of F. M. Alexander and Moshe Feldenkrais, and we danced and explored movement and other forms of creative expression. We also learned some anatomy of the skeleton and major muscles.

During that week I had two sessions with one of the teaching assistants. In those two sessions I sensed her attitude of open acceptance, both through her touch and through the way she spoke to me. Recognizing that this acceptance was what had been missing for me in my relationship with my mother, I experienced and expressed sadness. When not in class or personal sessions, I explored Greenwich Village with classmates, enjoying its shops, bookstores, and restaurants.

It was an incredible week for me, and by the end of it I felt very changed. As I drove home from New York with the orange light of the late-afternoon sun illuminating the trees in their mid-October glory, I reflected on many moments of the week and felt my soul illuminated by a deep joy. As I pulled into my driveway after the two-hour drive, my heart was overflowing with love for the world. I saw that my wife's car was gone and soon discovered that no one was home. Ordinarily, not being welcomed after a long absence would have triggered disappointment, but in this moment I felt joyful—full of joy to be home and to be alive. I took advantage of this wonderful opportunity to be home alone by walking in my garden. And it was glorious. There were still apples on the trees, and grapes and raspberries and wildflowers, and birds and smells and the beautiful sunset sky. After enjoying this bounty that was a part of my life, I went inside the house and drank in yet more joy as I sensed the abundance in my life.

Knowing the transient nature of all experience, I paused to wonder how long these wonderful feelings—this "high"—would last. And while I sat there musing, my wife and son came home. Liz came into the family room where I was sitting and gave me a big hug and kiss, sat down near me, and asked me how I was. I began to tell her, while opening a bottle of Bordeaux and filling two glasses. She listened intently and we savored our wine as I recounted some of the highlights of the week. She seemed so genuinely happy for me that I felt wonderfully supported. After several minutes our fourteen-year-old son, Jake, came into the room and with a cheerful "hi!" tossed his jacket onto the coffee table—knocking over one of the glasses and spilling the rich red wine across the tiled coffee table and onto the light earth-toned Navajo rug that was one of my favorite possessions.

Jake and Liz caught their breath, waiting for the explosion that was as inevitable as the rising and setting of the sun. But no explosion came! Instead I calmly said, "You go get some towels, and I'll get some club soda." Liz and Jake looked at each other in amazement for a few moments before getting the towels and helping me clean up the spill. The profound change from my usual reaction took all three of us by surprise.

They never really expected it to last. And to tell the truth, neither did I. I thought the mellow mood might survive a week or two before the old, familiar anger would return. But it's been over four years now and the calm, grounded feelings have grown. I rarely get angry. When I do, the anger is milder than it used to be. It doesn't build on itself, and I get over it much faster.

Since that first training week I've continued to work on myself, attending the entire three-year Rubenfeld Synergy training program and subsequent advanced workshops and trainings—all of which include receiving, observing, and giving sessions. My healing and self-understanding have continued to deepen. But it was that first touch—and that first session with Ilana—that I'll always remember.

My Body Suits Me Fine

Barbara McKenzie

I eagerly anticipated adolescence, when my chubby body would transform to resemble the figures of my two older sisters. It was easy for clothing to flatter their beautiful proportions. I dreamed of wearing their pretty clothes and looking like them. But adolescence brought a rude awakening: My form had been cast from a different mold. Short in stature and thick in waist, this pubescent cherub's proportions did not conform to conventional dress sizes, let alone conventional standards of beauty.

Disappointment and confusion about my body grew into self-loathing when new clothes never fit properly, despite Mom's creative alterations. Over time, thoughtless comments made by others and my embarrassment about how I looked in clothes took their toll on my self-image. I thought of myself as being large and overweight when, in reality, I was quite small, though with very different proportions from those of my sisters. Dieting didn't seem to help. No matter how thin I became, my "internal mirror"—like a fun house mirror—distorted my reflection so I still saw myself as grotesquely fat and much heavier and bigger than I was. My initially innocent diet and exercise regimens soon escalated into full-blown anorexia and occasional bouts of bulimia.

I recovered from these eating disorders twenty years later and, by early 1997, had been maintaining my weight and eating normally for fifteen years. The only trace of the past was my distorted image of my size and shape. Thankful for my recovery, I had no expectation that this misperception would ever change. After fifteen years, I believed it to be permanent. Then I encountered Rubenfeld Synergy.

As a student in the training program, I had many opportunities to increase my self-awareness. Of these, one stands out—the Rubenfeld Synergy BodyMind Exercises that started off each day. These subtle and delightfully relaxing practices awakened my curiosity and allowed me to explore at my own pace. One day, during a rest period between two segments of an exercise focusing on the hips, I spontaneously held my hips gently between my hands for several seconds. During other rest periods I felt my hips from different directions. Taking their measure in this way, I began to realize that I was not big-boned, as I had always believed myself to be. On another day my attention was drawn to my shoulders, and by exploring them with my hands I realized that they were not large, either.

I trusted this process of self-discovery and used my hands in many subsequent BodyMind Exercises to focus on other parts of the body. I became aware that my hands were operating as scanning devices, registering new and different images about my size and shape. I was very pleased with my new insights and after a while thought that I had used this new self-discovery tool to its limit. But a new variation of scanning with my hands brought me still greater awareness and understanding.

During one of the small-group training sessions, I was lying on the table as the "client" for a fellow student "Synergist" to practice on.[1] When she and the supervisor stepped away from the table to discuss something, I touched the top of my head with both hands. Then I did something new: I slid my hands simultaneously along the sides of my head and neck to my shoulders. As I connected one part of my body to another with my hands I saw in my mind's eye an outline of my head, neck, and shoulders—almost like the outline of the paper dolls I used to cut out as a child. And I *felt* childlike—playing, experimenting, and all the while learning about myself. My spirit was as free and light as a child's imagination.

In other practice sessions throughout my first year of training I continued to use my hands to connect parts of my body—running my hands from my shoulders to my hips or from my hips to the tips of my toes, and always visualizing the new parts of my paper doll outline. The experimental nature of the training supported my natural sense of curiosity. No one seemed to notice what I was doing. No one said anything to me about it. I appreciated the time and freedom to explore my body in these important learning experiences.

Through the touch of my hands, I was developing a new sensory awareness that integrated my individual body parts into a whole picture. I liken the effect of these explorations to developing a snapshot—from fuzzy negative to clear print. For the first

---

[1] Skills are practiced in small groups of four to six trainees under close supervision.–*Ed.*

time in my life, I had a clear image of myself. I was petite and slender after all—just as everyone had been telling me and as my small clothing size verified.

Not only was I seeing myself with different eyes; I was also feeling myself with a different heart. I felt a warm flush of love and appreciation for the gift my body was able to give me, and for how well it had served me. I saw and felt its beauty and was at peace. Now I truly know myself and am happy to say, "My body suits me fine!"

Transforming Wounds

INTO POSSIBILITIES

Lee McAvoy

I entered into the world of Rubenfeld Synergy while I was in graduate school studying to be a counselor. I became interested in studying some type of body–mind therapy to incorporate into my future practice. When a friend told me about a Rubenfeld Synergist in my area, I decided to have some personal sessions with her.

As I experienced my Synergist's light, gentle touch I had a sense of "coming home" to my body that was completely new to me. After just a few sessions, I noticed that in my day-to-day life my senses had heightened and my thoughts had clarified. I was more aware of my feelings and began to make more decisions based on what I truly wanted. At first these decisions were small, such as which restaurant to go to or what movie to see when I was with a friend. Yet being in touch with what I wanted in these moments was very liberating for me. I felt a confidence that was new to me. I was able to calmly assert myself and set limits with others, including people in authority and those closest to me, people with whom this had previously been difficult. For the first time in my life I was able to move through and beyond old habits of perfectionism and a persistent feeling of being overwhelmed.

Within a few months I met Ilana Rubenfeld. I sensed immediately that she would be my teacher and decided to enter the training. It was during my first year of training, in one miraculous session with Ilana, that I released childhood wounds and reclaimed my birthright as a writer.

The session began with a great deal of laughter as Ilana performed a mini Rubenfeld Synergy session on J. T., my blue stuffed bear. (Since sessions with Ilana were so in demand, I had reserved my slot by placing J. T. on the table.) I joined in the laughter and, sensing support and caring from the group, could feel my anxiety level dropping.

Once I was lying on the table, I felt her fingertips make light contact with the back of my head. I then experienced a gentle rocking as she placed her hands on my own, which I had folded protectively over my abdomen.

I felt Ilana's hands on either side of my left hip as she asked me to say a word or phrase or describe an image. The word *hallelujah* came to me immediately—most likely because we had just finished a conducting lesson in which Ilana had us conduct a rousing rendition of Handel's "Hallelujah Chorus." Ilana asked me to repeat "hallelujah" over and over, and we recited it together, like a mantra, as she gently swept her hands down the length of my leg and foot. When she asked me for a word for the right side, I chose to repeat the same word. Immediately my breathing deepened. I began to relax and let go of some of the fear I was experiencing. After she completed the sweeping motions on my right side, Ilana gently moved my feet; as she did this I felt movement rippling up my legs and hips, all the way through to my neck and head—a gentle pulsing through my entire body.

I became aware of Ilana's hands lightly kneading under my shoulders. Initially I felt tightness, then a great deal of warmth as the tension from my back and shoulders seemed to melt into her hands. Perhaps because I had already had a session with Ilana at a prior workshop, I felt safe enough with her to disclose the reason I had chosen to have this session—my feelings of guilt about having been unable, as a child, to prevent the sexual abuse of my two younger sisters by our paternal grandfather. Although I had recovered from much of the earlier trauma of his abuse of me, I remained plagued with guilt. Knowing intellectually that the guilt was unwarranted did not keep it from continuing or from interfering with my ability to use my creative talents as a writer.

Ilana identified these feelings as "survivor's guilt." Her listening, her words, and her touch were filled with compassion. I felt simultaneously accepted and deeply understood.

I told Ilana about the night before, when I'd had an insight while reminiscing with a cousin about our great-grandmother, who had died when I was three and my cousin was four. I have always remembered the last time I saw Nanny in the nursing home, suspended between Earth and the spirit world. At the time, my parents told me that Nanny was senile; but at three I had no trouble following the flow of her conversation. At one point she looked into my eyes and told me that she was giving me a pencil. This gift had a great deal of significance to me and I spoke of the incident with my parents many times, always telling them how much I yearned for the pencil. Being three, of course, I expected to be handed a real one. As I spoke with my cousin about this incident, I suddenly realized that Nanny, who was an artist who painted until she died at eighty-eight, had been attempting to tell me that I am a writer.

Throughout my telling of this story Ilana affirmed the power and beauty of the memory. I felt myself reclaiming my love for writing through my entire body. I also gradually began feeling a strong, visceral sense of innocence, and it became clear to me that the guilt that haunted me no longer served any purpose in my life. I said aloud that I was ready to release it.

To support my process of releasing guilt, Ilana asked me to create my own scene and method for letting the guilt go. I said that I would need "a big universe, lots of stars, and a big heart." I was also very aware of the presence of the spirits of four of my ancestors: Nanny, my maternal grandfather (who was very loving), my grandmother, and my Aunt Joan. I knew that they were there as spirit-allies and were very eager to assist me. I wasn't sure exactly how I would release the guilt, but I had complete faith that it would happen. I chose to begin by telling a story.

As I continued from "Once upon a time . . ." through the years of my childhood, Ilana sat at the head of the table, touching my shoulders lightly, sometimes on top, sometimes from underneath. From time to time I felt her hand over my heart. My story unfolded and for the first time I was able to speak—without feeling shame—of being nine years old, witnessing my sisters' abuse, being threatened if I told anyone, and feeling shame and guilt that I was unable to help them.

At this point I sensed that my guilt had settled—and was stuck—in my chest and abdomen. As I wondered aloud how to release guilt from my body, Ilana jokingly advised me not to send it through the mail. After laughing along with everyone else, I easily decided to let it flow out the top of my head and out through my feet. As Ilana gently ran her fingers through my hair, I could feel and visualize the guilt begin to move and dissipate. I experienced intense heat and shaking as an indescribable energy poured out through the top of my head and the bottoms of my feet. As both of us verbally reaffirmed my innocence, I was fully aware of the support in the room, from my spirit-allies and from the universe.

Although over fifty people (my training group and the teaching staff) were present for this session, I had a sense that I was enclosed in an infinitely large bubble of safety created by Ilana's unconditional love and regard. I felt simultaneously very visible and very protected—safe to go wherever I needed to go in the session, without being led or having to go there alone.

I also felt and sensed the support of the group through their tears and laughter during the session, and I received unwavering support from them throughout the remainder of the training week. The telling of their own stories, their compassion for mine, and our deepening friendships opened me to new levels of intimacy in my life. A deep calmness stayed with me for several days.

Once I returned home I began to make many internal and external adjustments so that my life would reflect my new, guilt-free state of being. Coming to terms with this new identity was somewhat disorienting, as I became aware of feelings that had previously been masked by guilt—fear, anger, sadness, even great joy. I made a wholehearted commitment to my writing, changed jobs, and let go of friends and situations that were sabotaging my well-being. Gradually the disorientation subsided.

Since then my life has continued to be enriched in numerous ways I did not even dare to consider before. My job is much more fulfilling, and my current friendships are mutually caring and supportive. But, since life is a process and not an end result, at times I still struggle. Sometimes I forget that the integration process is more subtle than just having moments of insight and letting go. When I become discouraged I open my eyes to see that because of a particular insight, I have altered my way of being in the world. I realize that I am whole and free, despite hard times, and I credit myself with the ability to love and care enough to implement positive change in the face of obstacles that once seemed insurmountable.

My session with Ilana showed me that if I am willing to release the burden of silence, it is possible for painful emotion to flow through and beyond me, as it did before the traumatic experiences of my childhood. Although I cannot completely determine outcomes in my life, I can be fully present for the experience of living and, thus, make optimal, life-affirming choices.

As a Rubenfeld Synergy practitioner, I use this new ability to be fully present to witness my clients' journeys. I try to listen not just with my ears, but also with my hands and my entire being. My hope is to be with my clients in a full, non-judgmental way— and so invite them to be with themselves in the same way. Facing and transcending my own obstacles has given me an unwavering faith in the power of each committed client to discover, through attentiveness, her own healing.

Recently I had a dream that I was flying through the sky at dusk, shooting straight toward the moon, stars, and planets. I was unassisted, holding only a leaf and a few pages of my writing. I wasn't sure where I was going, but I was completely calm, knowing that I would find absolute healing. Suddenly there was a flash, and I saw an image I knew to be both male and female. The image entered my body and traveled through it, recognizing my pain. I knew that the healer was also the injured, the image both God and myself. I awoke feeling more peaceful than I ever have.

What I Learned in the Pauses

Meg Morris

I often feel the need to do a lot of talking in order to figure things out. So it surprised me that in the process of my own Rubenfeld Synergy sessions, some of my greatest discoveries came to me during the pauses—periods of silence when my own inner knowing can speak.

One such instance occurred during my Rubenfeld Synergy training, when I was serving as a client for Ilana's demonstration. The lesson wasn't a demonstration of Rubenfeld Synergy, where there is usually a lot of dialogue and the focus is the "client's" personal physical and emotional work. Instead, this was a demonstration of a new somatic skill, a new way in which to use touch. Since this lecture was not going to be about me or my issues, I didn't expect to be doing much talking and, as I lay on the table,

I was aware mostly of myself—how I was lying on the table, where I felt tense, where relaxed, and where in between. I was curious but had no particular emotional agenda. Knowing that the trainees and teaching staff were seated in a circle around the three of us, I closed my eyes, feeling comfortable and safe.

This time, instead of demonstrating on me herself, Ilana chose to have Jos, one of my classmates, practice the new move on me under her guidance. Jos gently touched the sides of my head in the move we call "the first touch." Jos's hands greeted me lightly and respectfully, as if saying, "Hello, I'm here." It felt like an ordinary session, except that my attention was torn between enjoying it and following Ilana's lesson.

After the first touch Jos stepped away from the table, and Ilana asked him what he would like to do next. I tuned them out and went back to paying attention to what was going on with me, noticing as I did so that I was a little impatient to see what would happen next.

When Jos came back he touched the tops of my feet with his palms and then made contact with my soles—what I personally call "first touch for the feet." When he removed his hands my feet "twinkled" back at him. I felt some very young energy there, as if my feet were waving hello back at him.

From previous Synergy sessions I knew what would happen next. Sure enough, Jos's next movement was to assess the state of my pelvic area by moving my feet and ankles slightly with his hands. When he performed this movement I noticed that, as usual with me (and with many clients), my feet and ankles barely moved. I know that I tend to have a lot of tension or "holding" in my hips, and I felt ashamed that this part of me did not move as freely as I imagined it should.

What a coincidence, then, that Ilana said she would teach Jos a movement called the metatarsal spread, which speaks to the hip from the sole of the foot! Ilana began showing Jos how to apply pressure in a slow, steady, gentle pattern to the sole of my right foot. At one point I felt a ping! in my hip socket, followed by a rush of warm energy flowing back to my foot. I remember feeling my right ankle become loose and fluid in an uncharacteristic way, the way I imagined it should be.

Ilana invited me to comment on the difference that I noticed between my two sides. I paused, took a deep breath, and mentioned that while I was still holding a great deal of tension in my left side, with the foot pointed like a dancer's, my right side was loose and relaxed, with the foot and leg rolled slightly outward. I felt calm and peaceful and in a slightly altered, trancelike state.

And then, very calmly, I noticed that I was aware of this difference between my left and right sides without feeling that I had to fix or change the left side to match the right. For the part inside of me that has always striven for perfection and labored to "get it right," this was a great learning—and, boy, what a surprise! The gift for me was not only the experience of how relaxed and open I could be, but also that my relaxation was the result of a small, focused movement that "spoke" directly to the sole of my foot and indirectly to my hip and pelvis. It reminded me that movements do not have to be big or forceful to be effective. I also learned that indirect contact with my hip and pelvis, parts of me that have a long-standing pattern of tension, was a valid, if not better, way to say, "Hey! Will you let some of this go?"

Ilana and Jos then demonstrated the metatarsal spread with my left foot. For me the experience—of being there in my body and accepting my body and myself exactly as I was at that moment—was so new and so liberating that I just lay there, needing to do nothing else.

When it was time to end the demonstration I shifted to a sitting position and, after pausing, came to my feet. As my feet sank into the carpet I felt that I was making contact with the floor for the first time. As I walked I touched and explored the floor with different parts of my feet, enjoying the sweet and playful experience with the curiosity and wonder of a young child.

And then I rested. I had learned a lot about myself—how I usually am and how I could be—during the pauses in the session, when "nothing" was happening that anyone could see or hear. I was even "hearing" less than usual; in my semitrance, my usual internal chatter had quieted down. My body, with its own inner wisdom, didn't need talking in order to learn.

As someone who is "in my head" a lot and talks a lot, I am grateful for having had this experience. It was an important reminder that the answers will come for me if I ask the question and then give myself time to listen to the part of me that already knows the answer. And I expect that pausing will give my clients' inner wisdom time to provide answers for them, too.

Reflections

Annie McCaffry

I met Ilana Rubenfeld for the first time in London at the Festival for Mind Body Spirit in the early eighties. I was intrigued by her approach since I had by then worked for some years with both the Alexander Technique and past-life therapy. The subtle, safe way in which I experienced Ilana's work that day made me enquire there and then about the possibility of training with her.

"I can give you a roof to put all your learned skills under," she said. "But you must come to New York."

The training convened three times a year for three years—a format designed, I understood, to make it possible for foreign students to attend. Still, it was a heavy commitment of my time and money. I was married and living in London at the time, with three small children. As I prepared to travel to the United States for that first gathering, reluctantly leaving my beloved children in the care of my mother (who, I later discovered, feared that I had joined the Moonies and was unlikely to return), I was determined to get Ilana to do the second lap in the United Kingdom. I tried many a manipulative trick during that first stay to achieve my goal, without success. I clearly remember walking behind her down the corridor in No. 115 Waverly Place[1] on the last day, with her letting me ramble on until I had run out of reasons, whereupon she quietly turned around, looked me straight in the eye, and, with half a smile, said, "Annie McCaffry, you'll be here," and with that, she turned and walked on. "Yes, damn it," I thought, "I know I will."

Years later, after I had published *Journey to My Self,* Ilana told me she had felt that only if I were to get away from my Britishness and its influences would I be able to complete her training successfully. In retrospect I am sure she was right. From that training I brought home many immeasurable gifts, which are now deeply ingrained in my being.

One of the ways by which Ilana tested our awareness and sensitivity was to lie on her back on the massage table and invite the students in turn to stand at the head of the table behind her and place their hands either side of her head with the light touch that is such a stamp of Synergists. My turn came and, as my hands lightly touched her head, I heard her say, "Let go of your left knee, Annie." My heart leapt. How could she know through the touch of my hands what my left knee was doing? But she did, and today those I teach and with whom I work express amazement as I demonstrate that same degree of awareness and sensitivity.

Another invaluable gift came through Shirley Elias, one of

---

[1] The address of the Rubenfeld Synergy Center, where many trainings took place—*Ed.*

Ilana's former students, who was appointed to oversee my group of four students the day we had "outside clients" come in. "Risk all you can," said Shirley, "and if you have any problems, give me a wink and I'll get you out of it without the client ever knowing. This is your chance to push the boundaries of what you know."

"Hooray!" I thought, "I'll go for taking real risks." But as the story in my client's body unfolded with effortless ease, I assumed that he must be one of the easy, straightforward guys who didn't require any risk-taking on my part at all. "How disappointing!"— or so I thought until after the session was over and Shirley asked me how I would sum up my achievements. "I couldn't find a way to risk," I said despondently, "either by my questions or by my hands-on movements."

"What!?" she exclaimed in her strong Brooklyn voice. Her face a mirror of surprise she continued, "What are you saying? Why, the very way you brought him into the room was a risk! Not to mention how you suggested he lie facedown on the table instead of faceup!"

"Oh, was it?" I thought. "All I was doing was following my intuition and what seemed easy, natural, and obvious to me."

Back I went to England, where I already had a practice in body–mind integration, with the decision that if Shirley thought that what I had done was a risk I could easily risk trusting my intuition twice as much as I had that day. And that is what I did over the next two months. Whenever my logical mind gave a direction and my intuition said something different, I risked the latter. I had more and more fun with the success of this approach. Then back to New York I went for the final week of training, arriving full of excitement and eager to share, especially with Ilana, what I had explored and found out for myself.

In the opening session Ilana said that since we had learned the basic skills, she was going to show us how to take the work a stage further. And there, before my very eyes, she began to teach exactly what I had found out by my intuitive risking. That was it. I have never looked back since. The work has grown and grown, but now the focus has changed. I trust and follow my hands and my intuition, and my head follows, with the skills I learned always available to back me up.

Ilana added to my skills and gave me a roof for them all. I have travelled to many parts of the world to lecture and lead seminars, as well as do one-to-one work. I have learned that not only family but also racial patterns can be unlocked, healed, and transformed through this work, which continues to teach me new and ever more subtle approaches.

I would never have imagined that my practice today came from the blossoming of the scatter-brained Scottish girl from Auchtermuchty whom Ilana had courage and wisdom enough to risk inviting to join her Synergy training back in the early eighties.

When I published *Journey to My Self* in 1993, I realized just how much of its truth and accumulated wisdom I owed to Ilana's patience and insight. "I will teach you all I know," I remember her saying, "and each of you will take it and build on it in a different way and make it more." What a gift, what a teacher—not only of Rubenfeld Synergy, but of Life.

Seasoned by Celeste

Bill Miller

Sometimes I don't know what I know until I *have* to know it! This has been the case for me during my twenty-seven years as a portrait and architectural photographer. Over the years, I have learned to trust that no matter how many things go wrong on a shoot I can get the picture. When I began studying Rubenfeld Synergy, I expected the same would be true in this new field: I would "get it" when it came time to apply what I had learned.

In the second year of training we started to practice by giving sessions to volunteer, nonpaying clients. Ilana and the staff often told us, "These practice sessions are for you. Don't be surprised if your clients get value out of the experience, but that's not the main point. It's for you to learn." I wondered why they made such a point of saying this.

Eager as I was to practice, it was difficult to schedule enough sessions because I was out of town so often on photo shoots. To the rescue came my friend and fellow trainee Rachel,* who had more clients than she could handle and offered to refer Celeste* to me for sessions. Grateful, I didn't ask Rachel too many questions about Celeste, even when she said, "Celeste needs to be able to feel safe with a man; she has a lot to get out of her system."

When Celeste phoned to set up an appointment, I answered her questions about Rubenfeld Synergy and told her to wear loose-fitting, comfortable clothing. I didn't ask her much about herself, wanting to save that for the intake at the start of our first session. I have reconstructed the session here with the aid of my session notes as well as vivid memories of what I learned that day.

Celeste arrives five minutes early and rings the outside buzzer in an oddly aggressive way that makes me wish I knew more about her. She is the first practice client about whom I know nothing except her gender.

As I wait for the elevator to bring Celeste up I muse, "Why didn't I ask her more about herself? Or ask Rachel?" Then I notice myself getting curious about Celeste's apparent impatience and command myself to snap out of it. "Take a deep breath, Bill, and open the door."

I'm greeted by a woman I take to be in her early thirties. She is petite and demure, yet outlandishly dressed— sporting bright fuchsia hair, a very small halter top, and low-slung bell-bottomed trousers that reveal her bare midriff and the gold ring that pierces her navel. I am both puzzled and a little annoyed by this provocative outfit because I thought I had clearly described to Celeste Rubenfeld Synergy's gentle, respectful touch and the need for her to wear loose-fitting, comfortable clothing that would respect her modesty and my own.

Without making eye contact Celeste says "hello" and finds a seat. I review what we have discussed over the telephone and remind her that, as a student, I will be discussing our sessions with a supervisor. Keeping her head down, she quickly signs the release form as I continue asking questions. Is she taking any medications I should know about? Is she in any kind of therapy and, if so, does her therapist know about and approve of these sessions?

Her head seems to drop further. She has been on Prozac for a month and a half. For financial reasons she sees the prescribing psychiatrist only rarely. He has not yet responded to the message she left for him about our sessions. Celeste asks me if I can wait until next month, when she sees him to renew the prescription, for her to tell him. I tell her it would be all right.

Celeste keeps her head down during almost all of this intake and history-taking process. I am distracted by the incongruity between her shy demeanor and her provocative dress, between her soft, almost inaudible voice and her heavy hand on the buzzer.

Her story continues. She has recently returned to New York from Italy to escape her husband of nine years. She met and fell in love with him out west and followed him back to his homeland and family. He traveled on business, leaving her with his family, who seemed uninterested in her. Alone most of the time and hindered by not speaking the language, Celeste began to fill her time by baking. She opened a bakery, which brought with it prosperity, friends, and some visibility, as she and her bakery appeared on the evening news.

Her in-laws began to pay more attention to her, but

when her husband returned, he was upset by her new independence and self-confidence and almost immediately scheduled another long trip. While he was away she realized that their relationship was not good for her. When, upon his next return, he demanded that she move far away from the family, she decided instead to leave him and return to New York, which she did a year ago. She has just learned that her husband has located her and plans to come for her soon.

At this point in her story, I ask Celeste if she'd like to move to the table and continue her story there. It takes her a long time to settle comfortably on the table. I am grateful for the time because I need to settle in with myself as I prepare for the first, gentle touch of her head. Distracted by the many layers of her story, and the gaps in it, I remind myself to be calm, not to let my nervousness intrude in any way on Celeste's experience of being alone with herself in the accepting presence of a caring human being.

Calm at last, I approach the table and touch her head. Her first awareness is of a wall between her body and what she describes as herself. She tells me she feels safe behind the wall, yet she longs for what is on the other side.

When I touch her feet, my hands confirm the split she describes. Compared to the energetic buzz I felt at her head, her feet feel lifeless. At her hips, too, there is little energy. I am curious about this contrast and, after a while, decide to explore it with Celeste.

"Are you willing to do an experiment?" I ask her.

"Yes."

"Send the wall away on a long vacation, and listen to your body without the wall.... What messages do you get from your body?"

The first messages are all about numbness in her neck. She continues listening to her body and tells me that her neck is blocking her head from her body. After a while she describes a numbness in her back and says she thinks this numbness is about not being in touch with her heart.

I ask, "Is there a statement your heart wants to make?" After a long pause she says in a tiny voice, "I'm scared."

I mirror her, softening my voice and repeating, "I'm scared." Then, after pausing to let her continue being with her own thoughts, I continue, "What are you scared of?"

"Celeste can't take care of me, can't protect me."

As I gently place Celeste's hand over her heart I ask, "Is there anything you want to say to your heart?"

"I am really trying to take care of you," she whispers. I sense that the heart is only somewhat reassured. Celeste continues the dialogue, "My heart fears Celeste won't be able to stay away from him when he visits." As she says this her frightened whisper gradually grows into the voice of a petulant seven-year-old. "I can't take it. I can't go back to that relationship!"

Her tone of voice and a shuddering of her body give her statement a resonant vibration of truth. Suddenly Celeste bolts to sitting and almost growls with desperation, "I have to end this, this session. I've got to get out of here!" Then she covers her face, as if to hide her shame, and adds, "I have to run away!"

"What the hell do I do now?" is screaming in my head as I quickly review everything I've ever read, seen, or imagined about to how to handle such a crisis. Nothing.

Although Celeste appears ready to get off the table she stays there, eyes closed, sitting very still. Then an intuitive flash hits and I find my mouth saying, "You are free to leave the session at any time. And you don't *have* to."

She looks at me quizzically.

"You can leave and be alone with these feelings," I explain. "Or you can stay and continue in whatever manner you prefer. I can be a witness to whatever you're going through."

I wait. Miraculously, her breathing slows and her body relaxes as she seems to reflect on this. I continue. "It seems to me that your heart said it could never go back to that relationship, and the rest of you really felt the truth of it. I imagine that saying it out loud—perhaps for the first time—was very, very scary."

"*Pause, Bill, pause,*" I remind myself. Then, aloud, I repeat, "You are free to leave."

After a few moments Celeste lies back down on the table. She lies absolutely still for a while, sits up and looks me straight in the eye for a full minute, then lies back down.

"How do you feel now?" I ask, very softly.

"I feel less alone."

"Do you have any allies who can help you to reassure your heart?"

"I have my dog. I can't let my dog down."

"So, together you and your dog will make sure your heart feels safe as you face the visit of your husband."

As she agrees with this, she comes to sitting and looks at me again.

I reiterate how much we've covered for a first session and suggest that feeling safe in her heart could well be an ongoing challenge that she might choose to work on in future sessions.

"As you slowly come to standing, see how it is to be a bit more in touch with your heart."

Once Celeste is on her feet she walks around the room and marvels at the photographs she hadn't noticed when she arrived in such a rush less than an hour before, and says, "I missed a lot, keeping my heart walled up so safely."

When I'm photographing I do not think about, and rarely know, what causes me to trip the shutter when I do. Often I don't know what I've got until it is fully developed. Occasionally portrait subjects will ask, "How did you get me to be that way?" I do not have a good answer. They have recognized in their portraits aspects of themselves they had lost or longed for, or strengths they had been hiding from. I can't say where my resonance with subjects comes from.

I was reminded of this after Celeste's session, when I reviewed it before writing it up for my supervisor. I thought about the differences between photographing people and doing Rubenfeld Synergy. When I photograph people they follow *my* lead, trusting that I will tell them what to do to make them look their best. When I do Rubenfeld Synergy I follow *their* lead. I trust that their awarenesses will take them where they have to go. Instead of being open-eyed and alert, like portrait subjects, Synergy clients usually close their eyes and go into a semitrance. Despite these apparent differences, I realized there is a much greater similarity: Whether they're in front of the camera or on the table, I have to get out of the way so they can be themselves.

I finally understood why Ilana says these sessions are for us more than for the client. I felt that I had been "seasoned" by this session with Celeste. I learned that I can trust my sense of touch as well as my vision, and that not knowing is all right as long as I stay present.

BodyMind Exercises

Peggy Kostyshyn

By *the time* I was finally diagnosed with post traumatic stress disorder in 1989, I had been suffering for over thirty years from frequent, severe muscle spasms in my upper back and neck, resulting in incapacitating headaches. Nonaddictive medications were ineffective but, fearing addiction, I refused to take prescription medications. Four chiropractic adjustments a week relieved the headaches for short periods, but they recurred during my sleep and when I came under stress. I was in both individual and group therapy and had massage therapy twice a month.

I was still missing too many days of work as a discharge planning coordinator in an acute care hospital. Unable to control any aspect of my life, I was overwhelmed by feelings of inadequacy. Fearful of losing my job and income, I tried to compensate for my frequent absences by spending ever-increasing hours at work in a "workaholic" attempt to catch up.

In 1993 my sister visited me from Toronto, a two-day drive away. She showed me part of a Rubenfeld Synergy BodyMind Exercise that she had just learned at one of Ilana Rubenfeld's weekend workshops in Toronto.

> I followed along as best I could, lying on my side with both arms stretched straight in front of me at shoulder height. I bent my knees at a ninety-degree angle and kept my ankles pressed together as if they were glued. Satisfied that I was in the right position, I then mimicked my sister's small, slow, gentle movements. I slowly slid my top hand forward and then back a few times, repeating this until my arm slid easily. Then I repeated the same forward and backward motions with my top knee. Then it got more compli-cated—zigzagging by sliding my top arm forward and my top knee backward at the same time. After doing this on one side I stood up and walked around, feeling a profound difference between the two sides of my body.

I wasn't curious about the concept behind the exercise, but simply thought of it as another way of stretching my spastic muscles. And it did loosen them; I was so impressed by the results that I signed up for a weekend workshop the next time Ilana came to Canada.

At the workshop, after Ilana had introduced us to the philosophy and theory of Rubenfeld Synergy, she instructed us to do a simple exercise by ourselves:

1. Clasp our hands together with our fingers interlaced.
2. Notice which thumb is on top.
3. Take a mental picture of how this feels.

4. Release our hands and clasp them again, this time with the other thumb on top.

I didn't have to wait for her next instruction, which was to notice, because as soon as I clasped my hands in this nonhabitual way I felt a twinge of anxiety spread across my chest. I was taken aback. A mere change in the position of my fingers in relation to each other was causing me anxiety. I realized that it was not going to be as easy as I thought to stop having headaches simply by making certain changes in my body. I saw that the very changes I sought to make elicited the feelings I was struggling to reduce.

I was confused by this dilemma and approached Ilana at the break to share my experience with her. She smiled knowingly and told me that I had gotten the picture.

During the weekend, I was introduced to four complete Body-Mind Exercises. To my relief these did not bring up torrents of feelings, but only an increased awareness of my body, my posture, and my patterns of holding tension. I experienced significant changes from these sequences of small, subtle movements— changes that years of traditional stretches had not produced. I purchased a set of Rubenfeld Synergy BodyMind Exercise audiotapes to use at home and decided to apply for the next Rubenfeld Synergy training program with Ilana.

Hoping that learning more about the body–mind connection would speed my healing, I began to do the exercises at home. At times, feelings of grief or terror would well up in my gut, and I needed to slow down in order to allow them to emerge gently. When I pushed myself beyond my limit, I would quickly develop a headache. Learning to listen to my body helped me to accept and honor the mechanisms I had developed for self-protection. I gradually generalized this learning to other defense mechanisms of mine. For example, instead of berating myself for my perfectionistic tendency to demand too much of myself and others, I began to appreciate how that tendency had helped me survive my childhood. I even stopped shaming myself for "being stuck" in habits I hadn't been able to change.

I have had some remarkable flashes of insight while doing bodymind sequences—suddenly becoming aware of a new insight into an issue, a behavior, a relationship. One such insight was that although a certain person never listened to me—never even heard me!—I was still talking to him and expecting him to behave differently. Another was recognizing that I often play "Savior," feeling responsible for the whole world and trying to live everyone else's lives for them. No wonder I felt overwhelmed and resentful.

BodyMind Exercises are now part of my daily self-care routine, along with sitting meditation. Sometimes I skip the meditation and do several of the exercises instead. To me they feel like moving meditations. I also use specific exercises as soon as I become aware that my upper back muscles are tightening or when I am in emotional turmoil. Doing any of these exercises I almost invariably become aware of something I'm fearful about, and develop some new insight into it. The insight usually results in a speedy release of tension so that I can move quickly to the next constructive step in resolving the problem facing me.

During the weeks of training, we did a different BodyMind Exercise each morning. By doing these I learned to listen to my own internal rhythm and not push myself. I also heightened my awareness of energy moving in my body, which feels like my spirit coming home at last, leaving me feeling rich and full. Using the BodyMind Exercises has empowered me to take control of my own growing and healing.

I've Got To Be Travelin' On

Valerie Bain

Toward the end of my Rubenfeld Synergy Training, I did a piece of work[1] with Ilana that has greatly influenced the way I have lived my life ever since. I want to tell you about that experience as I remember it, with a little help from watching a videotape of the session made at the time.

I am not a procrastinator by nature, but I had put off asking for a demonstration session with Ilana out of shyness and fear of being the center of attention. Eventually curiosity overcame reluctance, and I found myself one afternoon talking quite comfortably with Ilana in front of the group and the camera.

Ilana put me at ease by reassuring me that I would not have to

---

[1] A demonstration session in front of the training group, so called because although it is a demonstration, it involves a piece of deep therapeutic work.

go any place that frightened me. I remember being curious and open to see what would come up in the session. I had no particular agenda for it.

Almost as soon as I lay back on the table I was jolted by the thought, "This feels like an operating room!" I didn't say anything, but kept trying to follow what Ilana was saying and doing. I became increasingly distracted. Something about the bright video lights above me and the circle of faces all around me was making me uneasy. Ilana noticed that my attention was not at my left hip, where I was attempting to make it go, and she asked me what was going on.

Suddenly noticing that my arm was outstretched as if it were attached to an I.V. tube, I told her that I had been triggered to memories of the operating room in which, six years before, both my breasts had been removed.

I was surprised by this reaction because, by now, I had fully recovered from the double mastectomy, emotionally as well as physically. The ensuing conversation with Ilana covered many topics: my not wanting my other arm restricted; my feeling restricted in life more by my own fears than by other people or events; even how brave I had or had not been, facing that surgery and others since. Ilana credited me with more courage than I thought was warranted.

After a while Ilana asked if there was anything else I wanted to say to my body.

I answered, "*You've* been through a lot, too!" and laughed aloud. As I continued looking to see what else I wanted to say to my body, emotions flowed through me. Tears came as I acknowledged, "I appreciate you." I felt strong as I said, "I'm taking better care of you."

Then Ilana asked if my body wanted anything else from me, something I should do or not do.

My sadness built and it took some time for me to be able to say out loud, "My body wants to hear that it looks all right....I know it doesn't."

"Where does your body want to hear that?" Ilana continued.

"Right here," I answered, touching my sternum, "at my chest."

For a while Ilana's hands rested on mine, which were crossed over my heart. I felt her lift them gently and then I felt them drop onto my chest, one hand on each breast. I laughed again, thinking, "Only Ilana would do that!"

Although I heard the group's gasps and laughter, I was not aware of being watched as Ilana continued, "What do you want to say to your breasts?"

"They're not real, you know," I answered, speaking to Ilana and not to my breasts.

Ilana asked me to say that again, which I did. Then, assuming the role of my breasts, Ilana asked in a cartoonlike voice, "What do you mean, we're not real?"

"They're better than nothing, but they're not real," I said. "They're comfortable. That's more important!" We discussed my earlier implants, which had been downright uncomfortable, and the possibility that my real breasts, off in a jar somewhere, were missing me after so many years of having been part of me. My feelings of gratitude grew as I recalled having nursed four children, and as I realized that in some sense, my breasts had sacrificed themselves so that I could live.

I told Ilana about a Canadian Cancer Society pamphlet that was given to me in the hospital right after my initial surgery. I'm sure that taking its opening words to heart helped speed my recovery: "You have had a life-saving operation." That's how I had thought of it. That's how I'd *had* to think of it in order to get on with my life. So, I hadn't dealt with my grief over the loss.

When Ilana asked me what I'd like to say to my "old pal"

breasts, all I could think of was the song "So Long, It's Been Good To Know Ya!" I laughed and everyone joined me in singing the chorus to the end, "And I've got to be travelin' on."

Ilana asked me again if I had anything else to say to my breasts. This time I shook my head and said, "No, that's all."

To see if this was so, Ilana checked my neck by pressing gently against one side of my head and then the other. My head moved easily from side to side; my neck was soft and loose, and Ilana commented, "Your body says, 'That's right.'"

Ilana then placed my hands onto my new breasts, saying, "We have a whole life ahead of us. Welcome to this part of my life," to which I responded, "And it will be quite a journey."

A while later, after I opened my eyes and sat up, Ilana had me look around at the group. Everyone looked pretty good to me—friendly and caring. The session became a wonderful celebration as Ilana and I walked slowly around the circle. Greeting each man or woman in turn, I felt a strong connection both to the individual and to the group as a whole. I felt as if I were participating in an ancient ritual, a celebration of the feminine.

My feelings of ease and lightness lasted for the rest of that training week. Then it was time to go home and continue to integrate into my life what I had learned in that session.

One major lesson was the most obvious one, that not grieving for my breasts at the time of the surgery—or afterward—had left a lingering emotional pain that would not heal on its own. I had done a lot of "griefwork" around other issues, such as the deaths, in quick succession, of several close relatives and the end of my marriage. I hadn't thought to mourn my breasts and my counselor at the time did not suggest it.

It took me longer to grasp a more profound lesson—that I'd be better off if I changed my old pattern of dusting over unpleasant things, pretending they're not there or will go away if I ignore them long enough. I had been doing that even at the beginning of the session with Ilana, trying to ignore the thoughts about the operating theater. Since that time I have become more likely to pay attention to my feelings, to attend to them at once. I notice sadness more readily, and express it. I also notice happiness more readily, and express that, too. Being more aware of my feelings also makes it easier to express them to other people.

Intention

Lee McAvoy

At the end of the first year, trainees
are required to demonstrate their
understanding of the major intentions
of the Rubenfeld Synergy Method.
Lee submitted this poem. —Ed.

In one hour
sandwiched between your life filled with right choices,
yet struck vacant, still, and empty without warning,
or for reasons we don't know,
you may come to me.

I welcome you, because I too have endured
that sunny day, unexpectedly shamed
and asking for help.
Words of compassion
and my invisible field of acceptance
tell you I care because I know self-care.

Your body's innate wisdom the vehicle,
we journey together

into a world of your creation.
You may feel momentarily God-forsaken
but possibilities will be born
from the silence hanging about in strips.

My hands, the youngest children
in awe and listening.
All senses open doors long nurtured.
My hands, the ancient teachers,
able to wait beyond eternity,
continue to pulse with faith and pride.

There's usually plenty to laugh at.
You can play mummy,
wrapping yourself in soundless strips,
peeking out with just your eyes.
Or, you can gather timelessness like wood
or flowers, reclaiming the darkest moments,
arranging an earthy bouquet.

As if witnessing the time just prior to
and the instant of birth or death
I am without escape route or magical cure.
Yet we will both become more fully alive, present,
and mysteriously empowered by all that unfolds
and the world-stopped places in between.

Together, when you are ready, we gather
buds of possibility. As your sacred witness, content
with all or nothing in my vision,
I give you yarn and string
while my hands and all of my eyes
become streams reflecting your truest image.

The Eye of Memory

Lydia Foerster

*Between 1994 and 1997, as official videographer
for the Rubenfeld Synergy Training Program,
Lydia Foerster videotaped over a hundred of
Ilana's demonstration sessions.*—Ed.

Today, I am the eye of memory.

I am hired to be here. To move with her moves. To look where
she points. To see the faces pinch or smile. To see feet twitch or
fingers flutter. To notice how they look at first, and then later. To
see how she stands, where she holds, how she works so that next
year and the year after, students will sit and watch and remember.

She touches and waits.

The muscles shiver and shift. Old ancient air—trapped,
entombed, held in stiff necks, bad knees—leaks out, stinking with
history. This is her witchcraft. To cradle heads and shoulders and
hip joints. To wiggle ankles until nerves and tendons, confused
and exhausted, let go with heavy sighs.

She asks the client, the trainees, me, "Is there anything you would like to say to your hip, shoulder, back, wrist?"

"Hmm...," we say.

The brow is furrowed at the thought of pain always there but never addressed so intimately, so affectionately.

The man or woman on the table—maybe twenty-five, or forty or sixty, maybe married with two kids, or divorced, or widowed— does something very strange. He talks to his hip.

"Relax," he says. "Stop hurting."

A steady thumb on the ball of the foot. She watches. She scans, I scan, the line: head-neck-shoulder-spine-thigh-ankle.

"And what does your hip say?" she asks, finally.

"Hmm..."

I have the best view. I stand in between, inside a circle of forty people who hang on the words and emotions, tears and twitches of the two in the middle. Moving, searching for a better angle, a closer picture, I am careful not to trip over cables or feet. I must think before I step—distribute my weight, ease my foot down, turn my head, adjust my shoulder, stretch my fingers, be smooth.

She waits with the strength of stillness, pauses, silence.

I breathe and the camera lifts and falls.

"It says...," he says.

And now I hear it, too, the breath behind me, sucked in, held, and in front of me the timid hiss of release.

"...it doesn't want me to forget."

She waits, then asks in a squeaky, childlike voice, surprised, quiet, "It doesn't want you to forget?"

"No, it wants me to pay attention."

And it begins. The face, eyes closed, reddens. Furrows rearrange themselves in various patterns of confusion and anger and sadness.

We hear stories. Fantastic stories. Of fathers who never said much and cars that came out of nowhere. Of young mothers who fly into rages when glasses are broken or suppers not eaten. Of grandmothers who tell secrets and brothers who laugh when sweaters are missing. And Mother is angry. Thirty, forty, fifty years later, Mother is still angry.

We are entranced, on the table.

I breathe and sigh.

Suddenly I am under the camera again. My face reddens and I cannot see the viewfinder. I close my left eye hard and press my right eye into the eyecup. I am the eye of memory, I say to myself. I shift my shoulders and check my focus. You are getting paid for this, so that next year, and the year after, eyes will see the things you have seen, the things they have missed or forgotten.

In the end, my right hand is stiff and red, my shoulders noticeably uneven. The muscles in my lower back are strained and my feet are sore. For days my face will be puffy and swollen with tears not cried for stories about people I do not know.

"I didn't notice you at all," they say, meaning even though I stood in between, there was only the table—and the layers of their own pasts peeled back.

"Thanks," I say.

Coping with Life

MOST PEOPLE who come to Rubenfeld Synergy as clients are seeking some kind of healing—physical, psychological, emotional, spiritual, or, most likely, some combination of these.

The following personal accounts illustrate the transformative power of the work. It is not surprising that many who initially came for healing have since decided to become Rubenfeld Synergists themselves.

Synopses

Wanting a Baby. Suzanne describes several months of work with Trish,* who is having difficulty conceiving.

Doing the Two-Step. Gilly and Paul's letters reflect their disintegrating marriage and the gradual changes that begin after Gilly's first week in the Rubenfeld Synergy Training Program.

Getting Out of War. Bineke is upset by the Gulf War bombing of Baghdad. As Ilana's demonstration client, Bineke relives a frightening memory from her childhood in Holland during World War II and gains a sense of peace and hope for the future.

Performance Without Panic. Mary, a concert singer, recognizes the source of her debilitating physical and emotional panic attacks. Building on this knowledge, she learns over time to manage these symptoms and her crippling performance anxiety.

Climbing Out of Depression. Carol's twin images of a snake and an iron rod reveal an inner resilience and creativity that fuel her recovery from lifelong depression.

Sexual Reawakening. Erica describes her work with Danny,* who has difficulty relating to women, and with Ellen,* who is uncomfortable with her femininity.

Learning To Mother. Carol's journey to fulfill her childhood dream of becoming a healer begins with her awareness that motherhood is bringing out the worst in her.

Mom, Alzheimer's, and Me. Tanzy describes how the skills she learned in Rubenfeld Synergy Training are helping her cope with her mother's Alzheimer's disease.

Wanting a Baby

Suzanne Forman

When Trish* first sought out Rubenfeld Synergy, she had been trying for a year to get pregnant. Her primary care physician was encouraging her not to be alarmed, as one year is the average time it takes for women in their midthirties to conceive. But Trish was distraught nonetheless, feeling increasingly depressed and overwhelmed. During our initial meeting, while sitting curled up tightly on a sofa in my office, she explained why.

She traced her despair to several sources. A close friend, Carol, had recently gone through what she described as "infertility hell,"

---

* Trish's story is based on that of an actual Rubenfeld Synergy client, with some features pieced together from other clients' stories so as to protect everyone's confidentiality while at the same time presenting actual case history material. While the details of these clients' histories vary, the themes are very much shared.

several years of medical workups, hormonal treatments, and surgical procedures. Trish, long mistrustful of doctors, dreaded the prospect of going through a similar process, especially since she knew the success rates of even the most technologically advanced treatments were modest, at best.

The strain was beginning to show in Trish's relationship with Malcolm, her husband of seven years. It had taken Trish three years to convince Malcolm to have a baby. Now she often wondered if she would have conceived more easily had they tried when she first wanted to. Her resentment toward him was increasing with each month's disappointment.

Worst of all for Trish was how she felt about herself: Her apparent inability to conceive triggered deep insecurities about her body and sexual adequacy. She was cloaked in shame, and saw her childlessness as a public advertisement of her failure as a woman. As these feelings grew increasingly difficult for her to talk about with family and friends, she became quite isolated. Deep inside she wondered if she was being punished by God for something she had done or failed to do.

Trish was brand new to Rubenfeld Synergy. She had enjoyed a few massages in the past and was a veteran of two successful psychotherapeutic relationships. When she'd heard about Rubenfeld Synergy from a friend, Trish was attracted to its somatic component and hoped that it might help her resolve her feelings about her body as well as offer her some comfort and a way through her desperation.

As we talked Trish gradually began to unfold on the sofa, and the lines in her face relaxed. I asked her, "How does it feel to talk about all of this with me?"

She breathed deeply and replied, "It feels good. This is what I think about all the time, and when I hear it out loud, I understand why I'm so stressed! I mean, it's hard to talk about, but I really need to. I can't keep this all to myself."

Hearing all that Trish had to say was an important part of laying the ground for our work, especially since she was used to talking about her feelings and trusted this form of communication.

I invited Trish to lie down on the table only in the last few minutes of our session, explaining that our goal was simply to begin to get to know one another through touch. She would get a sense of me as I made gentle contact with my hands at her head and feet, and I would get a sense of her as I listened through my hands. I suggested that Trish close her eyes, to give more of her attention to herself and what she was feeling. I relaxed my own body, cleared my mind, and approached her with curiosity and without judgment. As I gently touched her feet I asked myself, "Do my hands feel welcome here? How does Trish want to be touched? What does her bodymind have to say about her today?"

After a few minutes of this nonverbal communication, I invited Trish to open her eyes and share with me what the experience had been like for her. "It's nice not to think for a while," she said and, smiling shyly, added, "I feel like a little baby myself."

I asked a few questions to clarify what being a baby felt like to Trish. The baby state seemed to be a return to her essential self, when all of her fears about the future and judgments of herself and her husband were suspended. Perhaps as she learned to access that state, new possibilities would arise for easing her despondency over her childlessness—possibilities that she was not capable of recognizing in her current state of despair.

We agreed to meet weekly. In the next several sessions, in order to help Trish refine her body awareness, I began asking her questions like these: "Which parts of you feel more comfortable than others? How does your left side feel, compared to your right side?" I listened to her answers with my hands as well as my ears. Whenever there was a lack of congruence between the two, I'd gently bring it to her attention.

For example, one time as she lay on her back she described her neck as feeling open and loose, yet the muscles were so tight to my touch that they prevented any side-to-side movement of her head. I asked her, as an experiment, to tighten her neck muscles as much as she could. After a few seconds she began to laugh and said, "I see what you mean! I can't tighten them any more than they already are!" As her laughter subsided I again gently touched her at the base of her skull and, with my hands, invited her head to roll from side to side. This time it did, and she was able to feel the difference between her neck's new softness and its previous rigidity. This awareness of what her body was doing was very new to her.

Gradually we began to make connections between her physical state, her emotional experience, and the larger context of what was happening in her life. Despite some occasional softening, Trish mostly held her head exactly in center. I was very curious about this tightness and control, and, as a way to introduce Trish to a broader way of experiencing her tight neck, I shared with her some of the questions it had sparked in me: Was there some relationship between looking only straight ahead and not seeing other options? Was there something about being future-oriented or goal-focused to the exclusion of what was happening around her in the present? What would she experience if she did risk turning her head? How did this posture affect her ability to interact with other people?

Even though Trish didn't have ready answers to any of these questions, she became very excited at their implications. She expressed her appreciation that Rubenfeld Synergy was helping her come up with questions that were right for her and allowing her to listen for the answers over time. She said she would not feel comfortable with an approach that relied on a "quick fix" formula or that explained everyone's tight neck in the same way.

One of the first sessions in which Trish was able to tap into her body's wisdom focused on her legs. We had begun the session in our customary way, with Trish lying on the Synergy table and mentally scanning her body to notice how she was feeling, listening for anything that called for her attention. I was gently touching her here and there, feeling for anything that stood out to me. When I got to her feet, I jiggled them slightly and was surprised at the total lack of resistance I felt—all the way up to her pelvis, where her legs rolled loosely in her hip sockets. Because this amount of mobility was unusual for Trish, I was curious to see if it held a deeper meaning for her.

"How do your legs feel, Trish?" I asked.

"Really loose, unusually loose."

I moved to her right side and, with one hand under her hip joint and the other on top of it, cradled her hip between my hands. "Bring your attention in between my hands here, and tell me what you feel inside," I suggested.

After a long pause, Trish said, "Nothing. It's empty. The only thing I feel is the warmth of your hands."

I slid my hands down her entire leg and out past her foot. I then lifted her right leg and moved it around, still feeling for, and not finding, any resistance, nor any sense of Trish.

I made an intuitive leap. "I get the feeling that I could move your legs around in whatever way I want to, Trish. Does the sense of someone else having that ability over you mean anything to you?" I gently lowered her leg to the table so that her knee was bent and her foot was "standing" on the table. Then I cradled her left hip between my hands.

Trish took a sharp breath and her eyes welled up with tears. "Yeah, yeah," she said softly. "People can do anything they want with me. I'm really losing myself lately, especially with a few people who, I feel, are taking me over."

Trish's description of herself fit what I was feeling in my hands —an absence of substance and energy. I bent her left leg so that both feet stood on the table. They wobbled there until her knees leaned against each other for support. I placed one hand on each knee to heighten her sense of herself, and silently communicated to her legs that they could move or not move in whatever way they wanted to. Her legs remained still, propped against each other. Trish continued to speak.

"Remember my friend Carol, who had such a hard time getting pregnant with Jared? She has started asking me a lot of very personal questions—like what day I expect to ovulate, what position Malcolm and I use for making love—I mean very private stuff. I think she actually marks her calendar with my answers, because right about when my period is due, she calls daily, asking me whether or not I've started to bleed! It feels terrible to me, yet I always just give her the answers. I hate her for asking, and I hate myself for being such a wimp. I know she's just trying to be helpful, but I feel I have no right not to answer. What's happening to me?" The tears spilled out of the corners of her eyes.

I suggested, "Let's go back to your body. What gets your attention right now?"

"Well, I can feel my legs, though they still seem pretty empty...."

Her legs felt to me as if they were just beginning to wake up. "What else?" I moved to the head of the table, sat down, and placed both hands underneath Trish's head. Here, Trish felt very solid, warm, and present to my touch. Then I slipped my hands underneath her shoulders, which were also very receptive, though somewhat tight. Her breathing was rapid and shallow.

"It's my belly," Trish said. "It's as tight as a fist. I'm definitely holding onto something there."

"All right, let's check it out. What does that fist want to do or say, Trish?" I asked. "Let it speak."

Trish took a deep breath and responded. "Stop asking me questions! It's none of your business when I'm ovulating! You're invading my space! It's none of your business whether or not I've gotten my period! I don't want you to be the first to know if I am pregnant! Give me back my privacy! Go away!"

Trish's legs trembled as waves of energy moved down them. Her chest was heaving from her heavy breathing, her skin was flushed, and her shoulders were suddenly hot to my touch.

"What else, Trish? Let the fist talk to Carol."

Her voice came from deep in her body as she continued. "I'm really mad at you! I don't ask you to tell me about every time you have sex! I don't ask you where you are in your cycle! You make me feel like a bug under a microscope. Like a freak! You, of all people, you should know how I feel! I just want to be normal!"

I urged Trish, "Say that again, 'I just want to be normal.'" As she repeated it several times, she began to cry. Her shoulders softened dramatically. Gradually the tears stopped, her breathing slowed, and the waves of energy in her legs subsided. I asked her to check in with her legs and see how they felt as I gently rolled and cradled them.

"They feel heavy," she said sadly.

They felt heavy to me too, dense in a way that was new. "You sound so sad, Trish."

"I was just trying to think of the last time I did feel normal, the last time I had fun. I keep trying to remember the last time Malcolm and I had fun together, but I can't."

I suggested that she bring her attention back into her legs and see what was there now to be expressed to Malcolm, or Carol, or anyone else. My hands rested lightly on her feet. It took her a while to find a voice there. When she found it she said, "I need you. Carol, I need your friendship. But I need it to be different from the way it is now. And Malcolm, I need your love and support. I'm tired of being angry at you all the time. I hate that our relationship has become nothing but work. I hate that we don't make love for the pleasure of it anymore. I hate that I've cut you off from me as much as I have. I feel so sad, and so alone! I want to play with you, to be light, to feel close to you like I did before this whole thing started!"

Trish's countenance had totally changed. Her face had softened and was glowing. I rolled her head gently from side to side. Slipping my hands beneath her shoulders, I found softness and a strong presence. I returned to her legs, gently lifting and moving them, and felt changes there, too, which Trish confirmed. I asked, "Can you imagine actually saying any of this to Malcolm?"

"Yes, yes I can. He's going to welcome it." She grinned.

"Is there anyone else you'd like to say it to?"

"I think I just did. I mean, I needed to say that to myself."

As my relationship with Trish developed, I made sure to be authentic with her and let her know when something really fascinated or perplexed me. When my hands got information that differed from what she verbalized, I simply told her and then asked if my perception rang true to her. Just as I, as Synergist, can feel the truth in my client's body, my client can feel my authenticity (or lack thereof) as it is transmitted through my hands.

In later sessions Trish continued to experiment with setting boundaries in relationships with Carol and others. She began to share more of herself with Malcolm and to let go of her resentment toward him. I gave her the names of several therapists, and she was delighted that Malcolm was willing to go. There, in couples therapy, they began to learn new ways of communicating that helped them rekindle their love.

Trish also began to rely more and more on her body, and its inner wisdom, for guidance. When she was in doubt about what to do or say, she would check with herself for an inner sense of rightness. She waited until she felt the physical relaxation, the sense of knowing, the "yeah, this is right" voice of truth.

Several months of Rubenfeld Synergy later, Trish came in with some exciting news. She was pregnant, after nearly two years of trying! We continued to see each other regularly for a while and have now begun to taper off our sessions. I will always wonder whether or not our Rubenfeld Synergy work helped create the conditions that made conception possible. While this and similar experiences with other clients provide no definite answer, when I ask my own bodymind whether Rubenfeld Synergy is capable of creating a fertile environment, I get a resounding "yes." I am inspired to continue the exploration.

Dancing the Two-Step

Gillean Thomas and Paul Valiulis

Canmore, Alberta
February 25, 1996

Dear Paul,

I am trying to understand what has happened to us....

Before I met you six years ago, I was an independent woman. I loved the outdoors and was a fearless hiker, climber, rafter, and skier. I worked my way through university. I worked with young offenders and with Inuit in the Arctic, where there was total darkness for four months of the year. I loved adventure and travel. I trusted my abilities and my choices in life and that made me feel free and independent.

When we met in Mexico—on the side of Popocapetl—I was attracted to you from the start. I loved the twinkle in your eye and the conversations we had and two-stepping together in the desert.

However, since you were American and I was Canadian, I expected it would remain a platonic relationship. But every time you had time off from work you'd drive fourteen hours to see me in Jasper. When we married a year later, I thought you shared my sense of adventure and love of the outdoors, and were committed to our relationship forever. I trusted my choice to marry you.

Right away, your flings started. Sometimes when you came back from a trip, I sensed that you'd been with someone else. But when I'd question you, you'd deny it. My intuition was screaming at me, "Yes, he is!" and you were saying, "No, I'm not; what is your problem?" I felt I was going crazy. I lost confidence in my instincts. Finally, when I was six months pregnant with Tekarra, the truth came out. I was devastated, angry, and hurt. When I tried to express my anger, you said that the affair wasn't my fault; it had nothing to do with me. You said you'd never be unfaithful again. I wanted desperately to believe you—with a baby on the way, I had left my teaching job and we were getting ready to move—so I stayed in the marriage.

Since the move to Canmore, Tekarra and the new house have kept me busy. You have kept your promise to be faithful, but my trust—in myself and in you—doesn't seem to be recovering. I am still shattered by the memory of your flings. I sense that we are shutting down to each other, slowly but surely. When I ask you to spend time with the family, you berate me. I feel that whenever I want to talk, you close off—you give me a look of disdain and retreat behind your computer. Marriage counseling and individual counseling haven't helped. Things just seem to go from bad to worse. You walk in with a smile, and as soon as I look at you, your smile vanishes. I feel frustrated. I know how good we can be together, but it isn't happening. And even worse than feeling that I'm losing you is feeling that I am losing myself.

What really gets me mad, though, is how you show no interest in something I've found that sparks my interest in a big way—Rubenfeld Synergy. This is what I've been looking for since I was a teenager. Working as a counselor and teacher, I was always a bit frustrated, sensing that much more was going on with people than they expressed in words. This woman, Ilana Rubenfeld, practices and teaches a method that gets to the core truth for each person, and focuses on the practitioner's well-being as well as the client's. I appreciate that a lot. I haven't even experienced the work first-hand, yet I'm sure this is what I want to do for the rest of my life.

When I told you about her training program and my intention to apply for it, I was fully enthusiastic. I expected you to be supportive because I've supported you in your training to become an accredited mountain guide, and I've tolerated your long absences during your guiding trips. And I expected you to support me because I'm so passionate about doing this work. Your response to me was dismissal: "We don't have the money. You can't go unless you find another way."

Having always worked to pay my own way for my education and travels, I found it super-hard to ask for financial support from anyone other than you. Since you weren't willing, I shared the information—and my enthusiasm—with my parents and yours. Mine offered to lend me money for tuition; yours agreed to lend me money for airfare. Man, am I pissed off at you for not even trying to support me on this one!

I'm writing now because I just received notice that I've been accepted into the training program. It starts in a year. I'll try to hang in here with you until then. I'm hoping that when I'm pursuing my thing and satisfying my urge to travel and learn, then we will all be happier.

Here's hopin'!

Love,

Gilly

Canmore
June 17, 1996

Paul,

I can't take it anymore. You're normally not violent. When you threw the lamp into the wall last week, I bolted. When I returned and saw the mess from the lamp on the floor, it seemed like a symbol of our marriage—you make a mess and I clean it up. I'm tired of cleaning.

I do not want to talk to you now. Tekarra and I are going to Jasper. You can contact me there if you want to. I need space.

Gilly

Canmore
June 25, 1996

Gilly,

I'm sorry that you left and that we're so far apart. As much as I loved you in the beginning—and still love you now—you have truly been a bitch goddess from hell. Yes, I betrayed you and hurt you immensely at the start of our marriage, and for this I am deeply sorry. My intention was never to hurt you, but I was so caught up in the dysfunctional trance of my own sexuality that I didn't think my indiscretions had anything to do with you. I was wrong and you let me know it…again and again and again, *ad nauseam*. No matter what I did or said, it was never enough. I felt constantly hounded and harassed about almost everything, but what wore me down the most was hearing over and over again how "fucked up" I was. According to you, I am the source of all our problems and until I get myself "fixed" nothing is going to get better.

Paul

Jasper, Alberta
August 2, 1996

Dear Maggie,*[1]

Wow, the universe has really supported this move! I've left Paul and moved back to Jasper. It was a sudden decision, and on the drive up—between fits of sobbing—I wondered what I would do for work, child care, and a place to live. Well, within a day I had my own awesome place to live, which is next to impossible in Jasper. My dad's rafting company offered to train me on the Sunwapta River, so I have a new, fun challenge—guiding on a wild river. Yahoo! My mum and a girlfriend are looking after Tekarra, so I'm relaxed about who she's with. Whew!

I thought that spending the summer back home in Jasper would give me some space and possibly help my relationship with Paul. It hasn't helped. We just fight on the rare occasions we see each other. I'm usually out when he comes to see Tekarra. It's hard being a single parent, even with all the help I have, but it's still easier than living with Paul.

You know that training I applied for? I went to a preliminary workshop with Ilana Rubenfeld—the woman who developed the work and the training program. I was finally going to experience the work and be with the woman who'll be my teacher for the next four years—but I was so absorbed in grieving the end of my relationship with Paul that I was hardly aware of her. I spent most of my time alone. It was such a gift to have that time by myself to start to heal.

Then something neat happened with Ilana. We had this exercise where she had us all wandering around the room imaging someone who we were aggravated at. I was thinking, "'Aggravated'? Man, what a stupid word—I'd be aggravated at someone

---

[1] Gilly's best friend (not her real name)—*Ed.*

inconsequential, like the postman. I am pissed off!"

Ilana said: "Gillean, who are you aggravated at?" I burst out with, "'Aggravated'? I'm not 'aggravated'! I'm pissed off!" My story with Paul spilled out. Ilana "listened" to my body with her hands and said to the group, "Her body matches her words." That was such a relief to hear. My body relaxed when I heard it. All these years I believed I shouldn't be angry at Paul. Here she was saying if I'm angry, I'm angry. It's so, it's okay.

My story triggered a reaction from another woman, who was having trouble breathing. Ilana asked one of her helpers to stay with me while she went to this other woman. I was so absorbed in my anger that I was oblivious to the changeover. I *am* angry. Paul could never hear my anger, so I just stopped being angry— or so I thought. I didn't really stop; the anger was still there, only I didn't know it. I left him partly because I felt so much stress in my body from being around him that I was afraid I'd get sick— maybe even get cancer. Now I'm enjoying being angry and being able to express it to someone. I can see that if I hadn't worked so hard at swallowing my anger, it wouldn't have hurt me so much.

Mags, it is so lonely sometimes. I feel like my heart is being ripped out of my body. I miss having a man in my life, but I feel too raw to be interested in anyone. I also miss my house and my gardens. I made a magical flower bed this spring, before I left, and every morning I'd go out and say hello to my flowers. I made some human friends in Canmore, too. Now it seems so far away.

As time passes and things get easier, I feel that I'm finding myself again. I don't regret leaving Paul—only the way I did it.

Thanks for listening to this blah, blah, blah—that's how I'm feeling right now—blah. Maybe I'll be more cheerful next time.

Love,

Gilly

Jasper
December 15, 1996

Dear Mags,

Merry Christmas and a happy 1997!

I was lucky again and got another job just as the rafting season was finishing. I'm a liaison between families and the schools. I like it a lot but will be happy to have some time to myself when school breaks for the holidays.

Paul has been giving me enough financial support that I have to work "only" three days a week instead of five. That's a pleasant surprise! He always seemed like such a tightwad with his money.

We are also able to be civil with each other now—no more ranting and raving. I'm in my own life and feel quite separate from him. I've seen a lawyer about divorce, but neither of us is at that point yet. I wonder if it's just because Paul doesn't want to pay the legal fee. Sigh.... For me, I can't envision being with another man yet, so what's the point of a divorce? I'm already a single woman. I feel that in my heart. Heart is more reliable than a piece of paper.

Paul is coming to Jasper to spend Christmas day with Tekarra. He has been good about being a dad to Tekarra under the circumstances, driving the four hours from Canmore every chance he has to spend time with her. I'm glad he's making the effort.

I'm heading to NYC soon, for the first week of my Rubenfeld Synergy Training. Tekarra will stay with Paul and his family while I'm away. Talk to you when I'm back.

Love to the family,

Gilly and Tekarra

February 22, 1997

Wow, Maggie!

I'm on the plane—on my way home. This training is more than I ever dreamed it would be. I had three sessions during the week with Marisha, my Synergist for the year. Pretty intense! In the first session my "chronic" lower back pain vanished. I've had it for the past two and a half years, ever since I had Tekarra by C-section. I always figured that it was because my stomach muscles had been cut. But no, it was the experience of being physically and emotionally cut off from Tekarra at that time. Marisha and I replayed the scene so I could communicate and tell Tekarra that she was okay and not to be scared of the knife. What blows me away is that I was so unaware. All I knew and felt at the time was lucky—that I had a beautiful baby girl and that both of us were healthy! When I got off the table at the end of the session, my back pain was gone. And it's still gone! Pretty wild stuff.

I also had the exquisite experience of having Ilana work with me inside the healing circle of all 44 trainees plus staff. I'll share with you what I wrote in my journal.

I feel so connected to the ground and aware of how pleasurable that feels. Walking and sitting feel so different...and comfortable. I am aware of the world in a different way— the beauties of the world—joy and laughter. I'm noticing changes—the light on a bald man's head. Colors and eyes. Taking in the good things. Letting myself miss Tekarra and my mother and not blocking that pain of missing them. By letting them into my awareness I also remember how they look, and the joy I feel with them. I like this reality shift.

Talk to you!

Lots of Love,

Gilly

Jasper
February 25, 1997.

Dear Paul,

I observe that I'm smiling, and I imagine that's because I have an image of your face in my mind's eye. My body is discovering where it feels the pleasure of being. I am recently returned from the Big Apple. I love the training. I learned a lot—a lot about me. When I listen to myself—what's really inside of me—I want to love you. All those years, I was trying to get you to listen when all I really had to do was listen to myself. I'm now aware that I have choice. I can be angry with you—or I can love you.

I don't want to get back together with you. I want space to appreciate my experience, and the opportunity to integrate it into my life—in Jasper, just Tekarra and me. Love you, yes. Be together with you, no. I'm happy in my life in Jasper. I'm finally content to allow myself—and you—to be.

Lots of Love,

Gilly

Canmore
March 15, 1997

Dear Gilly,

I'm happy and thankful that you're training to become a Rubenfeld Synergist. The change in you has amazed me and I've fallen in love with you once again. This "new" you is wonderfully like the woman I met in Mexico years ago. I had forgotten how beautiful you are when your face is open and loving rather than angry and spiteful.

When you came back from New York after your first training session, the anger in your eyes was gone and I saw love for the first time in a long time. I actually enjoyed being with you and I now come to Jasper to see you, too, not just Tekarra.

Rubenfeld Synergy is a bit of a mystery to me, but there's no doubting the changes it has effected in you. I'm fascinated, and I want to experience this Synergy thing for myself. What are my options?

Love,

Paul

Charleston, South Carolina
May 5, 1997

Dear Gilly,

How's your life? Mine's a bit different these days. I went to see a Synergist on my way to South Carolina. I had an evening lay-over in New York and, after getting lost on the subway, just bare-ly made my appointment. A short while into the session I became nauseous and had to go to the bathroom to puke. By the time I walked down the hall and into the stall, the feeling had mostly passed and I wished I could have just let her rip into a bucket by the table. The sick feeling was something I felt I needed to express. When I got back on the table, I experienced my hips as being sad. "It's okay to be sad," I told my hips again and again. I opened my eyes and repeated this to my Synergist. In a flash I saw my mom and was telling her, "It's okay to be sad." This was her sadness I had taken on as my own. I cried until the end of the ses-sion and felt awesome afterward.

South Carolina was great. We played golf almost the entire time and on the last day I hit a hole in one. My dad hit a six-iron off the tee. On a whim, I borrowed his club. The ball flew, landed, rolled toward the flag, and disappeared. We all whooped it up after that, and I felt really good. The whole trip was good—I felt very open and secure in myself. That old family dynamic didn't seem to bother me that much. I'm glad I went.

Love,

Paul

Jasper
May 20, 1997

Dear Maggie,

Well, you know I told you about how I was feeling after my first week of training? Get a load of this: Paul was interested in my experience in the training. So he booked himself a session with a Rubenfeld Synergist in New York on his way through to visit his family. Anyway, he has come back a changed man.

We're not getting back together—in case that is where you thought this was leading—but his Synergy session did something to him. He seems more open and willing to talk, less defensive. I feel that I'm no longer a pain in the ass, but someone he enjoys spending time with. We're talking, and talking—it seems like there isn't enough time in the day! We're laughing, and allowing each other to be. Pretty funky!

Love,

Gilly

Quito, Ecuador
June 20, 1997

Dear Gilly,

How are you and how is your life? I'm writing to tell you about a very vivid and disturbing dream I had last night. In the dream, I'm driving with Tekarra in her car seat after having a bitter conversation/phone call with you. I'm driving recklessly, and Tekarra is somehow thrown out of the car still strapped in her seat. She's seriously hurt and I'm horrified at what I've done.

Slowly I realize that this is a metaphor. My recklessness is my desire for other women, driven by the conflict and misunderstanding between us. This recklessness will result in my throwing away Tekarra, seriously hurting her and me in the process. I don't want to do this. I want to understand why I'm reckless, and stop.

I'd like you and Tekarra to move back to Canmore so we can live together and work things out.

Love,

Paul

Canmore
September 10, 1997

Dear Gilly,

I'm relieved by how easily we reconnected, living together this summer. I know that I still have a lot of "stuff" to work through, but after working with a Synergist for a grand total of only three sessions, I also know how easy it is to get this "stuff" out of my body and start letting what I want to happen simply happen. I feel like I've been gently guided out of some of my "holding patterns" and have used my power to end this trance of mine and start feeling again.

I know that you, Tekarra, and I would not have this second chance at being together again as a family if the dramatic shift in you hadn't occurred....As it happened, the changes that brought us together again happened in both of us.

I love you, Gilly, and I want you to love me with all my sadness, strangeness, and happiness intact.

Love,

Paul

Canmore

November 3, 1997

Dear Maggie,

Sorry I haven't written for so long. Paul and I are back together! We've been together since June. I stayed and worked as a raft guide this summer in Jasper, and Paul was mountain guiding out of Canmore. We talked about where we would live. It felt easier to move to Canmore for this year, and see how it works out.

There was a perfect transition—Paul went to a five-day workshop with Ilana at Hollyhock. Tekarra and I went, too, and we all had a wonderful time. I still shake my head about how our relationship is now. We talk, and we are quiet together. We laugh, and we cry. We have the occasional disagreement, and the next day it's gone. I don't hold on to things anymore. I also allow myself to get angry when I feel it. And I allow myself to love and laugh. It's wild that it's so different. I am listening to me.

Love to listen to you, too—write back soon.

Love,

Gilly

Getting Out of War

Bineke Oort

In January 1990 I found myself in a war again. This time I was among the fortunate, sitting at home watching it on television. Presumably, I was safe. But was I?

Watching the people in Baghdad being bombed, day after day, stirred something deep within me—a pot filled with strong emotions. I felt compelled to keep watching. I had a strange feeling of being home again, a strong identification with those who had to endure the bombings.

It wasn't just ordinary news on television. For me it was hauntingly real. I had been in the same situation as a little girl, living in the Hague, Holland. What about all the innocent children, women and men who were being killed this time, or being maimed or traumatized for years to come? From deep recesses of my body arose feelings of powerlessness, terror, and anger, together with a sense of deep despair. "What is happening?" I wondered. American soldiers, who were rescuers and heroes when I was a child, were now bombing defenseless people in Baghdad. "How could my friends do this? When will mankind ever stop the insanity of war?"

The Gulf War broke out on a Thursday. On the following Monday I left for New York for the second week of training in the Rubenfeld Synergy Method. I was so overwhelmed by my feelings of powerlessness and hopelessness about the state of world affairs that my efforts to become a better therapist seemed woefully inadequate. I was filled with negative thoughts: "So what if therapists succeed in helping some people heal and live in peace? What difference does it make in the greater scheme of things? Are we not just rearranging the deck chairs on the *Titanic* while the ship is going down?"

I arrived at the Rubenfeld Synergy Center hoping I would have the opportunity to heal my old war wounds. Each afternoon of the training, when it was time for Ilana to demonstrate a complete piece[1] of Rubenfeld Synergy to the entire training group, my anxiety would flare up. Should I volunteer to be the client? Or should I just let it ride? One day I hinted to Ilana about my torment but I couldn't make up my mind or muster the courage to volunteer. Fortunately, I was saved from having to decide, because numerous cotrainees eagerly volunteered to get on the table.

On the last morning, when we were preparing to reenter the world outside, Ilana looked at me with a chuckle on her face and asked, "Well, Bineke, how about it?" I had no time to consider the invitation. Flustered, I climbed onto the demonstration table

[1] Unlike demonstrations for the purpose of teaching specific somatic techniques, these "real" sessions explore personal issues.—*Ed.*

ready to do my work. It was time to place my war-wounded "inner child" on the table, into the sensitive "listening hands" of Ilana.

An incredible hour followed. Looking back, I can best describe the session as "getting out of war." With infinite patience and gentleness Ilana led me to reexperience being in the war, while making it feel safe enough for me to enter and remain for some time in this dangerous, fear-filled place.

We focused on one recurring situation: standing in the basement of my home, covering my ears, and waiting for the dreaded roar of aircraft overhead and the thunder of their exploding bombs. Ilana accompanied me back into my time and place of terror. With calm presence she coached me through a reliving of the experience of covering my ears so as not to hear the next bomb. My spine shivered and I heard noises inside my head.

"Bineke, breathe," I heard Ilana remind me calmly. When I focused on my breathing, the noise in my head disappeared and the sense of terror and confusion ebbed away. For a short while I felt calm. But the next flood of strong feelings followed almost immediately.

This time it was not fear, but rage—rage at those now in power, for leading us into war once again. Overwhelmed by feelings of powerlessness, I began to rant and rave at the leaders of the world for continuing the violence of warfare. With her gentle hands and soothing voice, Ilana kept close contact with me while I expressed my tumultuous emotions and thoughts.

In this state of heightened awareness, I saw clearly that world leaders do not have the skills they need for the nonviolent resolution of conflict. Once again my mind spiraled downward into a whirlpool of hopelessness. Despairing, I said, "If the current emphasis on armament continues, we'll never get out of this rut."

Ilana then invited me to do what in Rubenfeld Synergy is called "the experiment." She suggested that I take charge of designing the training for world leaders. What would my curriculum be?

My ideas started bubbling up. Emerging from my helplessness, I found I had several good ones. A required course in Rubenfeld Synergy was the first thing that came to mind, to get the leaders in touch with their own emotions of powerlessness and vulnerability so they would no longer have to act out by abusing power. Ilana let me meander through my brain-body. The next idea that emerged was gardening. By working with and in nature, I thought, students would learn much more about the natural processes of cooperation than by studying only in indoor classrooms and libraries.

In my imagination I designed a "garden of the world" that incorporated many types of flower gardens—French, English, Oriental, a desert garden, and more—all blooming next to each other in perfect harmony. A new world was taking shape here, a world of color, beauty, and peace. A new world to feel at home in, a home for the soul.

As so often happens in this synergistic process, Ilana had the perfect tool to support me on my inner journey—away from the ugliness of war and toward beauty and harmony. She invited me to open my eyes. When I did, I found myself looking at a magnificent color photograph of a pink orchid. The warm, shining colors penetrated deeply into my soul. There followed a banquet of the most beautiful color photographs of flowers I'd ever seen— a bright red anthurium, yellow gladioli, red roses, and many more. I feasted my eyes and drank in the nectar of all that beauty.

Later I heard that Ilana just happened to have those photographs in her collection. When I began to describe my gardening curriculum, she quietly asked one of the training assistants to fetch the photos.

The session affected me so deeply that, later in the day, I felt able to reenter the everyday world with a renewed sense of hope and optimism. The war outside was still going on, but inside me there was peace. A new lightness of being began to overcome the shadow that had been cast within me so many years ago.

For a week afterward I was unusually aware of my breathing and other body pulsations. Somehow I knew that vital life energy had been freed within me. Feeling empowered by this new energy, I realized that the Rubenfeld Synergy Method was a true gift: one that would enable me to help others to heal, just as I had been helped to begin my own healing process.

Performance Without Panic

Mary Hopkins

Like most people I didn't really think much about my body unless I had an ache, pain, or illness, or unless I noticed something I wanted to change for the better. Then, in my mid- to late thirties, some of my aches and pains became more persistent.

I developed troubling and elusive medical problems—some benign, others potentially serious. I experienced a host of strange neurological symptoms that were eventually diagnosed as a type of migraine called "classical migraine." I was also concerned about the onset of high blood pressure and heart rhythm disturbances. In visit after visit to doctor after doctor and specialist after specialist, no concrete causes could be found for my combination of ailments.

In the same time frame, I began working with a therapist in an

231

effort to confront chronic anxiety and periodic panic attacks, which had troubled me off and on for years. The panic and anxiety manifested themselves in many parts of my life, but they were most upsetting when they intruded on my work as a professional singer and musician. With more intensity and greater frequency, performance anxiety was progressively crippling my ability to perform in public, and even my ability to sing in private. I could not understand the peculiar nature of this fear. Standing onstage I would be fine—until I heard the music leading up to my entrance. Then my heart would pound and my mind would race and every shred of my carefully cultivated classical vocal technique would evaporate. When I opened my mouth to sing, instead of sounding like a polished professional, I would sound like a scared child.

My experiences in conventional psychotherapy were very positive. It became apparent that the anxiety had its roots in events of my childhood—events I had thought had been long since resolved. Apparently not. Despite the considerable progress I was making in conventional therapy, dark, inaccessible places of the spirit remained. I was at an impasse, feeling that I had more to do, yet not knowing how to move ahead. I felt anxiety about the present and fear about the future, especially about my body and my seemingly declining health. Frustrated and saddened by my inability to overcome the performance anxiety, I began to sing less and less.

My therapist suggested body-centered work and Rubenfeld Synergy in particular. She explained that sometimes a mind–body approach can be particularly helpful when exploring emotional issues that have their roots buried deeply in the past. I had heard that traumatic experiences could be "held" in the body—that somehow our bodies remember the things that have happened to us even when our minds don't appear to. I had no strong opinions about these concepts. Feeling neither gullible nor skeptical, I simply kept an open mind as I made my first appointment. Little did I know that I was embarking on a life-changing adventure.

In the early sessions Beverly,* the Rubenfeld Synergist, would have me lie on the padded table with my eyes closed. When she asked me what part of my body I was most aware of, it was usually around my chest, heart, or midsection. I began to think about "heart phrases"—"matters of the heart," "hard-hearted," "soft-hearted," "fainthearted," "lionhearted," "coldhearted"—and how they were significant to me. I also began to think about how I had come to know my own heart in recent years—racing, pounding, thumping, and frightening me. I had never thought that events from my distant past might be affecting my heart (and me) so profoundly in the present. Was it possible that my heart had a story to tell? I was determined to find out.

In one session I lay on the table with my eyes closed, as usual. As I focused on my midsection and heart area, I began to feel very uneasy. Vague and disturbing feelings started moving in me. As Beverly encouraged me to keep my awareness focused on my body, it seemed as if a Pandora's box of sensations had opened. I saw images and visual fragments that didn't make any sense to me. Beverly asked what I was seeing, feeling, hearing, smelling—all the while reassuring me that I was safe. My uneasiness increased to the point where I wanted to open my eyes and stop whatever was going on. Knowing that I *could* stop the session anytime I wanted to, I felt safe enough to continue a while longer.

I began to smell a rotten and vaguely familiar smell. It reminded me of a person I once knew. Then, in a moment I shall never forget, the jumble of unrelated images assembled themselves into a place I remembered, and my uneasiness became a full-blown remembrance of a time and place of justified dread. There was music in that place, too. Twisted into the deep love I'd had for music, even then, was a memory of imminent danger—

and a knowledge that the danger came from someone associated with music. My heart raced, pounded, thumped, and I realized with absolute certainty that my body's current reactions were identical to my panic at that time long ago. I felt myself trembling all over.

Later in the session Beverly placed one hand under and one hand over each shoulder and hip joint in turn. For each joint she asked me to gather, in the space between her hands, any thoughts or feelings that I wanted to get rid of. Then she ran her hands down my legs or arms. After she did this with the first arm, I felt lopsided. It was as if one arm were light and free, and the rest of me were hung with weights. The feeling of release was so powerful that it startled me. After she finished contacting all four limbs my entire body felt physically lighter, and my mind unburdened. When I sat up I felt strange, as if I were inhabiting a different body. My mind felt strange, too. I was full of questions about what had just happened. I was surprised when Beverly suggested not analyzing the experience but rather "living with it" for a while. I remember telling Beverly that it felt as if I had been rewired or something. She smiled one of her wise smiles and said that, in a way, I had.

I thought about that session many times in the following days. I was astonished that I had relived the emotions and sensations of the past so vividly. All I had done was focus my awareness on a place in my body and allow the memory to surface. I thought with new insight about how and why my body tended to overreact with relatively little provocation. I saw that my body had programmed its reaction to danger long ago and continued its pattern of responding with "code red" intensity whether a danger was real or perceived. It was a stunning revelation.

After several years of Rubenfeld Synergy, I look back with wonder and gratitude at the discoveries it has brought. Over time and with lots of work my panic attacks, performance anxiety, migraines, and heart symptoms have been greatly reduced. I am especially pleased that I am able to sing again. After a recent performance a longtime friend said, "You must record those songs. You are in peak form."

When I experience an occasional increase in symptoms, I regard them as allies rather than enemies. They remind me to look for the cause, and sometimes they even give me clues about where to look. Almost always I discover some event, circumstance, or interaction that has triggered the habit of fear I knew so well in the past.

My experience with Rubenfeld Synergy helps me to live in the present with greater ease and understanding, and to face the future with anticipation rather than fear. Difficult times are far fewer now and are infinitely more manageable when they do occur. I am now aware of the strength of mind, body, and spirit that has always existed in me. I am able to appreciate my new insights and draw on them, thanks in part to Rubenfeld Synergy and the support of a gifted Rubenfeld Synergist.

Climbing Out of Depression

Carol Smith Ali

As a young child I dreamed of becoming an orchestra conductor. Although I loved music and took piano lessons for six years, I didn't have enough self-confidence to pursue my dream. I spent almost every summer at the family compound, surrounded by cousins, aunts, and uncles who I thought were much smarter, wittier, and more creative than I was. By the time I reached my teens I was spending a lot of time thinking, "I'm not creative," "I'm not fun," and "I can't express myself." I felt as if a dark, stagnant cloud surrounded me.

Two of the strongest beliefs I'd inherited from my family were "It's important to be self-reliant" and "Seeking help for problems is a sign of weakness." As a result it was a long time before I thought of reaching out and asking for help.

In my early thirties, after losing a lot of weight and energy in a single two-week period, I was diagnosed with a stress-related hernia. My physician prescribed Valium, which seemed to alleviate the symptoms. The Valium also gave me a foggy feeling of well-being. Several years later, when I read that Valium was addictive and destroyed brain cells, thereby creating memory loss, I decided to stop taking it.

A different physician supported this decision. He said I might be depressed, and suggested that I start jogging to raise my endorphin levels and reduce my dependence on Valium. I took his advice, but it was not easy to let go of this seven-year addiction. While tapering off I experienced fear and anxiety attacks that were intensely physical and real. I just kept exercising, jogging, and breathing through the feelings until they dissipated.

Six months later I had left the Valium behind. But my "black cloud" was still there. Taking Valium had merely covered up my underlying inner pain, just as aspirin may take away headaches without eliminating their causes. Finally I acknowledged that I needed to seek help in exploring some dark places. I started to read about depression and worked with two psychotherapists for several years. The insights I derived were often interesting and thought-provoking, but they did not penetrate my body or change my self-perpetuating negative thoughts or behavior.

Then one weekend I attended a holistic expo in New York City, where I saw Ilana Rubenfeld give a workshop on the body–mind connection. Although I was attracted to the gentleness of Ilana and her work, it wasn't until seven years later that I realized I wanted to explore this work for my own healing. After having several powerful sessions with a local Synergist, I knew I wanted to become a Rubenfeld Synergist myself and entered the training.

The turning point in my recovery was a series of sessions in which I made contact with a creativity I hadn't realized was in me.

The first glimpse of this creativity came through images and metaphors that developed in response to my Synergist's gently touching and "listening to" my body. I remember one session in particular.

My left side brought forth the image of a snake and my right side brought forth the image of an iron rod. At first I was startled. Where did these images come from? What did they mean? Initially the snake frightened me; I have always been afraid of snakes. However, I felt intuitively that this snake was gentle and feminine. In the dialogue that developed during the session, the snake told me that I could glide with ease and flexibility through the metaphoric grasses—the challenges—of life. The iron rod spoke sternly, from a fearful and rigid place. "Don't bend," it commanded me. "Fight; keep up your defenses and protect yourself." No wonder my right side and shoulder were so often stiff and in pain—I'd been lugging around an iron rod for forty-five years! In that session, under the Synergist's gentle hands, much of my tension gradually released and the unyielding rod began to soften.

Over the course of several sessions my right side became increasingly open and flexible, my left side more contained and focused. I felt as if both sides were working together and exchanging qualities. I became aware of the connection between my creative, gentle, feminine energy and my more masculine, active, take-charge energy. I felt centered, balanced, and powerful, and began to manifest aspects of myself I had long kept hidden.

Most exciting was my new ability to find meaning in these multifaceted images and appreciate the rich color and vibrancy of my psyche. As each session presented new and different images to explore, my excitement and creativity increased. Even my nightly dreams became sources of thought-provoking imagery. In place of familiar feelings of flatness and boredom, I began to experience the richness of possibility within me. I became more interesting to myself—and to others.

Each time I returned to New York for a training week, some of my classmates would comment on changes they saw in me— how much more lively I seemed, how much stronger. My sense of humor resurfaced. Of course, I wasn't the only trainee to change. Gathering together only every three or four months made it easier for us to notice changes that we might have missed if we saw each other more frequently.

The images that emerged in my sessions often connected me to strong emotions from my present life and, more significantly, from my past. Where there had once been a dark and dismal void, I began to discover hidden feelings—sometimes of anger, fear, and sadness, and other times of peace and joy. As my Synergist and I worked with the events beneath each uncovered emotion, new layers of creativity and aliveness emerged. I no longer felt stagnant or stuck. My depression was gradually pushed off "center stage" into the background, and finally disappeared along with my old habit of negative self-talk.

Having spent forty years in depression I relate easily to clients who are depressed. I find it spiritually rewarding to help them connect to their own energy and creativity.

Each of us has emotional scars to heal. Even if the scars are similar, each person's path to healing is unique. One client's message from her family was that she had to be still and quiet. The gentle, slow movements of Rubenfeld Synergy awakened her dormant ability to move gracefully. She took up interpretive dancing and learned to integrate feeling and movement into her life. Another client had been afraid as a child to express anger toward his violent father. Instead, he had turned it destructively onto himself. Through our Rubenfeld Synergy sessions he learned to give safe expression to his rage, to channel his energy positively, and to take responsibility for his life, both personally and professionally. Several depressed clients had learned at an early age to repress all spontaneity in order to be "good." Rubenfeld Synergy provided them, as it did me, the opportunity to recontact lost feelings and creative energy.

Life threw me a few curve balls in the form of low self-esteem, illness, and depression. I am grateful that I was able to take these balls and run with them. By exploring my feelings and inner resources I moved away from harmful family beliefs toward my own healing path, which led me to the exciting realm of touch and talk. From this exploration I have gained a new sense of awareness, balance, power, and success in the world.

This is my gift from Rubenfeld Synergy—connecting past experiences and feelings with present body sensations and images. Making these powerful connections was and is, for me, a lifeline to continuing awareness and change.

Sexual Reawakening

Erica Goodstone

Sexuality is an intrinsic part of our bodies and our lives. Men and women alike often crave the physical and emotional connection that only sexual intimacy provides. But for many of us, our natural sexual feelings and desires are frightening; sometimes we repress and hide them or make unfair demands upon our partners to satisfy our sexual cravings. When we are centered and loving we are able to accept ourselves as we are, including our full sexuality, and to allow others to be fully themselves. However, many of us harbor feelings of fear, shame, humiliation, anger, and even rage—feelings that often interfere with our sexual intimacy. Some of us even wish our sexual feelings would just go away.

In my Rubenfeld Synergy practice, many clients begin to confront and heal lifelong issues that have been interfering with their ability to become intimate. Danny* and Ellen* are clients whose problems with intimacy are quite common.

Danny

Danny phoned to find out if I could help him with his problem. "Women either reject me outright or they offer to be my 'friend.' I just want to love one woman and get married. To me sex is something you do in marriage. I guess it's necessary. But I think most women have had too much sexual experience. Why do they have to talk about it so much? Talking about sex makes me feel uncomfortable."

I reassured Danny that his feelings of upset and confusion about sex and intimacy are not unusual, that many of us have difficulty expressing pleasurable sexual feelings and that this can keep us away from close relationships. Sexual expression, I explained, is a natural part of life, nature's most powerful way of leading men and women to connect with each other, but certain early experiences can dampen our desire and make us feel guilty, embarrassed, or afraid of our sexual feelings. Rubenfeld Synergy, I told him, offers a way out of this problem by reconnecting us to the feelings and sensations that have long been held in our bodies. As we allow ourselves once again to feel our feelings, our fears of closeness and pleasure and sex gradually diminish.

Then I began to tell Danny how I work. I explained that in the first session I would take a detailed history, asking lots of questions and encouraging him to talk about his life, medical history, family, early childhood, relationships, and sexual experiences. In the following sessions he would lie down—fully clothed—on a padded massage table in order to receive gentle touch that is neither sensual nor sexual.

He asked, "How can this help my problem with women?" I explained my belief that our bodies hold the key to all the personal issues in our lives, including our sexuality. Receiving gentle touch therapy would assist his body to let go of habitual tensions, thereby making it easier for us to uncover and explore together the deeper meaning in his life. I wasn't sure Danny understood what I was saying, but curious and seeking help, he made an appointment for the following week.

When Danny arrived at my office I saw a frail, slightly balding, sandy-haired man in his late forties with shoulders hunched forward and a forlorn expression on his face. He greeted me with a limp handshake, as if he could barely muster the energy to shake my hand. I welcomed him and invited him to sit down. After we chatted briefly I reminded him that this history session was the only time I would take notes, and that the rest of the sessions would be a combination of talking and tablework.

Reviewing his life and his family history proved quite revealing. Danny's back straightened and his dark eyes darted back and forth as he recalled, "My father was always abusive to me and my two older brothers, as far back as I can remember. Mealtime was the worst because we hardly ever talked. We were all literally on the edge of our seats, afraid to say anything that might set off Dad's rage."

Suddenly Danny's eyes seemed to open wider and I could almost detect a smile as he continued, "But it wasn't always that bad. When my mother was alive she used to protect me. My brothers, too, but mostly me. I was the baby and her favorite. My brothers later told me that she rocked me in her arms when I was a baby. And when I got older, she brought me into the kitchen to help her whenever Dad got crazy. Trying to make sense of his crazy behavior, she would explain that he was 'just being a man.'

To me, 'being a man' was horrible. But at least I had my mother. I loved the smell of her cooking and the way she sat and talked to me about life."

Now his face took on a sad expression as he explained that his whole life changed drastically when his mother became ill, first with diabetes and then with heart disease. From the time he was eight, his mother was in and out of hospitals. After more than two years of being an invalid at home, she died just before Danny's eleventh birthday. During this period his father teetered unpredictably between severe depression and sudden outbursts of rage. "He took his frustration out on my brothers—and they took theirs out on me!" Danny exclaimed.

Danny told me about being beaten by his father and being teased and hit by his brothers. He had loved his mother and still loved women, but he didn't want to "be the man" with any woman. At the end of the session I reminded him to dress comfortably for the next session, which would involve tablework.

When Danny arrived the following week, I asked him how the history session had been for him. He said that it was the first time he had talked about his mother in a long time and that he had left the session feeling quite sad and had almost cried—something he hadn't done in many years. We conversed easily for a while about his current job, the blond secretary he often fantasized about at work—who seemed to give him mixed messages—and his lonely nights and weekends. When, during a lull in the conversation, I asked if he'd like to get on the bodywork table, his body stiffened.

I reassured him that this would be a gentle, safe experience and reminded him that I would not use touch for sensual or sexual arousal. I explained that the session was his—for reconnecting to his own feelings—and that if at any time he was uncomfortable, did not want to be touched, or did not want to talk, he would be free to tell me to stop, free to sit up, free even to leave if he wanted to.

Seemingly reassured, he removed his shoes and lay on the table facedown. Observing his position I noticed an unusually large, knotted muscle protruding from the middle of his upper back. His breathing was shallow and barely audible. Looking for other signs of tension or discomfort, I asked if there was anything going on in his body that I should know about before I touched him. He shook his head. Keeping his arms close to his body and his feet tightly crossed, he appeared to me to be tied up with an invisible cord.

Danny's body showed tension in other ways, too. For example, when I lifted his arm slightly and then let go of it, it stayed up in the air instead of falling back onto the table. In the first several sessions on the table, when I asked Danny what he was aware of in his body his typical response was, "Nothing." Over the course of several weekly sessions, his body relaxed more and he began to share more thoughts and feelings with me.

In one session, about three months into our work together, with my hand gently resting on Danny's hunched upper body I asked what he was experiencing. His immediate response was, "Tired."

I probed further, asking, "Tired of what?"

He answered, "I'm tired of working so hard to please people. Nobody seems to care anyway. I listen to these guys at work—they're so selfish and mean to their girlfriends...but girls seem to be always chasing after them, calling the office, showing up, buying them gifts. I just want to be with one girl, to take care of her, buy her presents, make a home together. But nobody wants me. I'm just a loser. My father always told me that."

"Aha," I thought. "Here's a possible opening, a personal belief that may contribute to his problem connecting with women." Making a mental note to explore this further at a later date, I continued the gentle touch to allow Danny to relax some more. Keeping my hand on Danny's back and continuing to observe his body for about five more minutes, I suggested that he might be more comfortable lying on his back and I invited him to turn over. He did so slowly and a bit shyly.

When Danny was lying on his back, his shoulders were so rounded and his chest so constricted that I felt a need to support his head with a pillow. In this position his arms were tightly crossed against his chest and his feet were again crossed at the ankles. His breathing was so shallow that it seemed to have practically stopped. His facial expression and body language appeared to me to be saying, "Keep your distance. Don't touch me. Don't hurt me."

Touching his head very gently with my hands, I felt enormous tension there, as if he were holding on. I encouraged him to see what it would be like to allow his head to rest in my hands, to allow his head to be heavy, to not to hold on to it so tightly. After a time I felt his head relax slightly in my hands and I noticed some softening of the expression on his face.

"I feel the weight of the world lifting off my shoulders," he said. "It's as if a dark cloud has been covering my face, not allowing me to see clearly."

Seizing this opening I asked him, "Danny, what is it you don't want to see?"

He blurted out, "I'm a man, just like my father! I don't want to be a man. I hate men! I hate being around them! …I like women better. But they don't like me."

I responded, "You've got a real dilemma. You're a man but you hate being a man. What do you hate about men so much?"

He quickly answered, "They're mean and they treat women badly. And they brag to each other. And they lie, and they get violent. When my dad acted crazy, my mother always reminded me that I was a man and I would someday protect a woman from men like my father. That terrified me! I never wanted to grow up. Nobody taught me how to protect a woman—how to be strong, how to fight—or even *what it meant* to protect a woman."

Toward the end of our first year of working together, Danny revealed a deep sense of shame about being male and having sexual feelings. One day he admitted to me that he had always hated his erections and had actually prayed for them to disappear. When he woke up from a wet dream or, worse, when he succumbed to his own increasing desire and masturbated, Danny would be mortified, ashamed, and angry with himself for not being able to resist. Locked in a state of internal confusion, depression, and imminent rage, he was tied up in knots of his own creation.

Danny's body held the key to these knots. As the gentle touch helped him to release the tension in his body, his images, thoughts, and memories came more readily into his awareness and some of his hidden feelings began to surface. Expressing his anger, sadness, humiliation, and embarrassment—and talking about those feelings—led him to understand more clearly the real sources of his conflicts with women. An often helpful exercise was to pretend that significant people in his life were in the room and to dialogue with them in a role-playing manner. In one such session he actually raged at his beloved mother.

"How could you have left me alone like that? You made me feel so safe and secure, so protected. You taught me that men were bad and you would always be there for me. And then you got sick and you ignored me. When you died I was all alone. Everyone else abused me. My body just closed up. I've been closing up around myself for years." At this point Danny motioned that he wanted to actually close up, so I guided his body into a fetal position and provided him with tissues as he sobbed quietly.

Although this was a real emotional breakthrough for Danny, it took him many more sessions to come to terms with having lost his mother at such an early age. In one poignant session he imagined hugging his mother good-bye, shrinking her into a tiny being, and keeping her inside his heart.

By the end of two years, the clump of tension in his upper back had noticeably softened. He had come to realize that this part of his body had been literally holding on to angry and hurt feelings since his mother's illness so long ago. As his invisible knots gradually released and unwound, Danny found himself getting angry, too, at many of the women he had cared for, who had only wanted to be his friend.

One time he exploded, "You just want to be my friend. I'm not man enough for you. Why can't you see that I need your help? I need you to protect me just like my mother did."

In that session he got it! He finally understood that he had been seeking and expecting women to replace his mother. In the next few sessions he began to forgive his mother for leaving him, then to forgive his father and brothers for not being more caring and supportive, and finally to forgive himself for having ruined his own chances to connect with women.

Toward the end of our third year of working together, as he continued to get more in touch with his issues, Danny began dating women again. This time he connected with women who wanted to be with him. He joked easily about his new problem—how to gently tell some of them that he wasn't interested in them. His posture was visibly more energetic and confident, and his solid handshake was evidence of his newfound inner strength.

Ellen

In her initial phone call Ellen complained of an inability to feel pleasure in her body, even in sexual relationships. During her first session she told me that she never desired or enjoyed sex and had never liked her body. For the first two years I saw her she wore mostly oversized beige or tan sweaters with baggy brown pants or long, pleated plaid skirts. Several months into our sessions, I commented about her clothing; she recalled that when she had begun developing breasts she would purposely hide her new curves with loose-fitting blouses, long, full skirts, and bulky sweaters.

Over a period of several months, Ellen developed an ongoing dialogue with different parts of her body, giving each of them a voice. By doing so she discovered that she had been ignoring the needs of her body for most of her life—her neck, shoulders, and lower back as well as her sexual organs. So great was Ellen's tension that the three times she had allowed herself to engage in sexual intercourse, she had felt only tightness and pain.

During one session I encouraged her to give her vagina a voice. At first she was embarrassed and found this a peculiar thing to be doing. After a while "Ellen's vagina" asked Ellen, "Why did you ignore me? Didn't you know I hurt? Why did you let those men get so physical when you hardly knew them?" During this session tears came to her eyes as she realized that her body belonged to her and it was her own responsibility to allow herself pleasurable feelings.

These insights marked the beginning of Ellen's long, slow process of change and integration. After a few months she started to take better care of her body. At my suggestion she took some long baths, during which she would touch her body in a loving, tender way. Afterward she would rub fragrant oils into her skin.

Her skin took on a more radiant quality, while her movements seemed freer and more graceful. After two years of Rubenfeld Synergy sessions she had eliminated junk food from her diet, was walking regularly and taking yoga classes, and was dressing in more stylish and flattering clothes.

As her connection to her body improved, she began to see herself as an attractive woman. She found herself becoming friendlier and less fearful of men. When she started dating again, she was not afraid of being touched. She was starting to enjoy her newfound femininity while knowing she could protect herself and be assertive.

My work as a Rubenfeld Synergist continually reminds me how we are all basically alike. With our chattering minds, our bodies clamoring for attention, and our spirits struggling to be heard, we are longing to be safe, secure, and loved.

Touched and heard without judgment or expectation, perhaps for the very first time, clients are able to observe how they think and feel, hear how they talk, and become aware of the "language" of their own bodies. As these clients open up to new possibilities—for thinking, behaving, creating, and becoming loving and sexual in the world—their lives often change dramatically. They begin to forgive themselves for those aspects of their personalities that have blocked their intimate connection with others.

As our work together nears completion, some clients even come to appreciate their initial problems—for having given them so much pain that they finally faced themselves and, in the process, became free to enjoy life more fully.

Learning To Mother

Carol Seewald

As a child I had a secret dream of being a healer—"secret" because I couldn't imagine how to achieve it and because I didn't know any "healers." I wasn't even sure what form this might take. Today I suspect that my grief over my mother's episodes of mental illness were at the core of this longing. Back when I was eight, I only knew it had something to do with helping people feel better. I didn't know it would take four decades for this dream to manifest. This is the story of the unfolding of my life quest and how I learned that healing begins within the healer's own heart.

Commitment to my personal journey began in earnest about the same time I became a mother. I had taken time out from my career in speech pathology to focus solely on mothering. I recognized that parenting "with awareness" was a challenging task.

Still, it surprised me to discover that my children, even as infants, were able to elicit emotions in me that were far more intense than given situations warranted. There were many times I was unable to contain or explain the tremendous riot of feelings I experienced. I felt unprepared for my new role as a mother.

From the start I took my babies' crying personally, as if it meant they did not approve of my ability to care for them. I felt overwhelmed at the amount of energy they consumed as I tried to keep them contented. When they weren't quiet or at peace, I felt I was failing as a mother. I remember crying right along with them on bad days. Occasionally I behaved in ways that reminded me of my parents at their worst. This frightened me, since I had sworn never to repeat their mistakes. One day in particular is etched vividly in my memory.

At 10:00 A.M. I was tired. Having slept fitfully the night before, I was already at the end of my emotional rope. It was during the early weeks of an unplanned pregnancy. My four-year-old son, Luke, was bored, and he amused himself by taunting his two-year-old brother, Ben. By the third round of shrieks, I snapped. I screamed venomously at them both to stop, and lunged at them in anger. Luke turned away and Ben gasped. Suddenly I noticed their faces. Terror.

In that single instant I knew they both felt their lives were in jeopardy. Time shifted. In slow motion I watched with horror as Ben choked down his fear and clung to me in desperation. He looked up at me with a pleading face that tore open my heart. I sensed he was completely willing to do anything in his two-year-old power to placate this monster I had suddenly become. His very life depended on it.

This desperate response jolted me out of my anger. Weak with shame, I collapsed, wondering how I had managed to lose touch with my responsibility toward these children, who were so dependent on my care. And it appalled me to have done something I found utterly abhorrent in others.

I could have dismissed this incident as just a bad day; after all, doesn't every parent have discouraging days? But I feared these episodes would intensify if I did not find out what caused the darkness lurking in my psyche. I embarked on a quest for a more peaceful way of living. Resolving to find better ways of handling my frustrations, I began to read voraciously. I had already been meditating for several years, and I began to explore different methods. I started keeping a journal and recorded my thoughts and feelings.

I also renewed and deepened my involvement in La Leche League, a self-help group for parents. I was grateful to have a place to go with my young children where like-minded people discussed, among other things, ways of avoiding hurtful crises. There I learned to communicate more effectively, as well as lovingly, and to develop more realistic expectations for both myself and my children.

As the early years of mothering passed and my youngest child began school, I joined a study group whose members came together weekly to meditate and discuss ways of living with greater integrity. We shared and pondered the richness of our dreams and learned how frequently we judged others, as well as ourselves, with critical hearts.

These new friends and I often compared notes about the various workshops and retreats we had attended. I was drawn to experience one in particular—a weekend-long workshop in the Rubenfeld Synergy Method.

There, within a short period of time, I was amazed to find myself moved, often to laughter or tears, as individuals shared stories of personal triumphs, tragedies and traumas. Somehow, within this safe container that Ilana Rubenfeld created, I could relate to the universal themes behind the stories—fear of embracing life more passionately, sadness about unrecognized dreams, and anger at the unfair abuse so many of us suffer in this supposedly civilized world. It was a relief to allow such a wide range of feelings to move through me. I marveled at the resilience of the human spirit and its capacity to attain greater integrity.

We listened as Ilana explained how "emotional holding" translates into physical holding, and, to illustrate this, we did slow, gentle bodymind awareness exercises. I was surprised to learn that the purpose of these movements was simply and profoundly to notice our bodies as they were, instead of trying to get them to move in some particular way.

Some of the simple movements had the unexpected and intriguing effect of bringing my emotions to the surface. For example, in one sequence we coordinated breathing with tightening the abdominal muscles for a sit-up only inches off the floor. Every time I rose up on the out-breath, I felt a wave of sadness. When I inhaled and came back down, the sadness was gone. The suddenness of this surge of emotion caused me to wonder if, at a physical level, my body was holding some unresolved emotions, just as Ilana suggested. It was a curious thing. My usual patterns— breathing in on the sit-up or holding my breath altogether—did not elicit this sadness. Only when using less effort to sit up in this new way, combined with breathing out, did the emotion emerge.

The most striking effect of the Rubenfeld Synergy workshop occurred upon my return home. Walking through the front door I discovered that, quite literally, my vision had changed and my perception of colors was enhanced. I was greeted by my children and my partner, Richard. As I saw their eyes, a spark passed between us—a joyous recognition that is beyond description. I simply knew bliss, right there and then. Everything sparkled with a clarity and brilliance I had never seen before. This unforgettable experience confirmed that the journey toward wholeness is neither intellectual nor predictable.

I may never be able to identify what it was about the Rubenfeld Synergy workshop that could have led to this bliss episode. Perhaps it was the unique combination of movement, humor, gentle touch, and listening. In any event, it strengthened my resolve to continue my search. I attended other workshops when they were offered in my area, and I began individual sessions in order to explore how my behavior had been shaped by traumatic events and how my mothering conflicts had their roots in my childhood. During these sessions the Synergist's gentle touch provided assurance and guidance as I reexperienced feelings of abandonment and fear that were still lodged in my body, ready to surface at the slightest reminder.

Along with these feelings came spontaneous memories. Some were both tender and painful—like the one of being a little girl watching my mother become very sick after the birth of my brother. By re-viewing that period from two perspectives—as a child then and as a mother now—I knew it had been a tragic time for my whole family. I was also able to feel the physical impact it still had on my body. Tears welled up abruptly and anger wrenched my heart.

I also had memories of sweetness and joy—like the one of a chaotic day when my daughter, Molly, was just weeks old. Between tending her and looking after the family's basic needs, there was no time for just sitting and enjoying her newborn beauty.

Knowing from experience how soon she would outgrow sweet infancy, I mourned. That night, in the wee hours, I awoke to my hungry daughter's fitful whimpering. As I put her to my breast for her night feeding I realized there were no phones ringing, no other children clamoring for attention, and no meals needing to be prepared. This was *our* time. I savored her newness, her softness, for a few precious moments, and a deep peace came over us as we snuggled contentedly back to sleep.

Often during my sessions physical sensations of my memories came to the forefront. Focusing on these sensations gave me a sense of internal movement. I could feel, for example, air going into my lungs as my chest muscles loosened and released tension. This in turn brought a corresponding shift in my emotions. While I had anticipated feeling the emotional impact of memories, I was surprised by the intensity of their physical impact.

Each memory affirmed, in one way or another, that both joys and traumas are a part of life—life in which babies are born and loved ones die. During times of stress I tended to act toward my children as my parents had toward me. They were the only role models I had. It was a legacy that would continue unless I was willing to change the pattern. My sessions with the Synergist gave me opportunities to express my strong feelings and practice new ways of responding to stressful situations—patterns that, over time, came to replace the old ones.

The relief and release I experienced in the wake of my sessions had a remarkable effect, particularly within my family. We learned to respect each other's boundaries and abilities to be self-responsible and supportive. For instance, one heart-numbing summer our Ben—then eighteen—was diagnosed suddenly with a brain tumor. The night before his surgery, Richard and I were able to honor Ben's wish to make out a will. It took all my strength to allow him to consider dying. Even though we later celebrated the success of the operation, my "mother-heart" will hold that anguish for the rest of my life. I know this event was also his rite of passage, his personal confrontation with death, his decision to ask his family for support.

Several years after that first workshop, I chose to embrace my dream of becoming a "healer" by studying formally. Ilana Rubenfeld's model satisfied my personal requirements for a gentle, non-invasive, and authentic method of enhancing awareness. I was comfortable with the fact that it is done with the client fully clothed. Most of all I appreciated its focus on the client, knowing that in my own case, healing and lasting personal change had emerged from within myself, not from some external authority. As Ilana has said:

> *The ultimate existential responsibility, as well as the moment-by-moment response-ability for change, rests with the client. The Synergist is there primarily to catalyze the change process, or in a musical sense to conduct it—or better yet, to serve as the guest conductor—but not to write the score or take the instrument out of the player's hands.... The live performance always belongs to the client.*[1]

My childhood aspiration has been fulfilled by my completing the Rubenfeld Synergy Training Program and practicing this profound healing work with others. It has been a long path, forged from the natural resources of my heart.

---

[1] Rubenfeld, I. (1988). Beginner's hands: Twenty-five years of simple, Rubenfeld Synergy — the birth of a therapy. *Somatics*, 6:4, 4–11.

I feel both the joys and the losses in my life more fully now. Each event, each person I touch, brings a distinct rhythm to my days. Feeling my body's reactions to these new experiences, these new contacts, gives me more options. I can cry when I am sad, laugh when I feel joy, and give voice to all the feelings my body holds. In my quest for a more peaceful life, I have learned that children as well as adults mature emotionally in the presence of a compassionate witness and a loving community.

Mom, Alzheimer's, and Me

P. Tanzy Maxfield

A year ago, following a series of tests, exams, and a CAT scan at the Stanford Alzheimer's Research Center, my mother Irene, my brother Bill, and I heard the diagnosis together. The doctors gave us the good news: "Irene, you are in excellent physical health." And the bad news: "Since we've ruled out everything else, you are probably in the early stages of Alzheimer's."

Though painful to hear, the diagnosis didn't surprise us. Only months before, Mom had been contacted by her eighty-three-year-old brother for the first time in seventy-three years. He told her that the two of them were the only survivors of the original six children, from whom Mom had been separated at age six. Three siblings had died from Alzheimer's and the fourth had died too young for it to have shown up. This contact with her brother intensified her sadness and sense of loss. At the same time, it comforted her to hear about her early childhood in Fitchburg, Massachusetts. He was able to validate the bits and pieces she had been recalling—for instance, "I was walking behind my grandmother and brothers and sister in the snow. They probably were breaking a trail in the snow, but I was so small and the snow was so high that I couldn't see anyone. I was afraid I would be lost. I've been afraid of being lost ever since."

A few years before Mom's diagnosis, I had realized that our relationship as equals—adult-mother and adult-daughter—would peak and then, because of her diminishing faculties, she would no longer be fully available to me or to herself. At that time we were enjoying a wonderful relationship through letters and occasional visits where we'd sit around her kitchen table, chatting and drinking tea or, occasionally, coffee laced with Kahlua. I snapped a mental picture and began to savor those times, knowing that they would not last forever.

In the fifty-three years I've known her, Mom has taken up canasta, cribbage, exotic egg painting, pottery making, photographing old barns, collecting decorative plates, sewing, gardening, sailing, gambling, fishing, trailer camping, and bird-watching. She has raised parakeets, canaries, and African violets. She has been a devoted sports fan, holding season's tickets for the '49ers, watching the Giants on television, and attending her granddaughter's soccer games. She has been widowed three times. She has held many jobs: dropping off bundled stacks of the Shopping News *for the young boys with bicycle routes; elementary school secretary; high school librarian; sales clerk—first in a plant nursery and then, after retirement, in a gift shop on the Boardwalk. She dreamed of driving a diesel truck cross-country.*

I had known there would come a time when our relationship would enter new territory, one in which neither of us had any training, modeling, or family experience. And now it was upon us.

Since her diagnosis, Mom's phrase "I'm losing my mind" has taken on new meaning. She really is losing her mind. Not going crazy, not insane, but losing those functions that allow us definition of ourselves, our history, how we got to where we are, and how we live our life day to day.

She knows what she's losing. She writes everything down to keep track of her day. When we talk on the phone she'll read her notes to me. She then describes what she sees out her windows— the birds, the trees, the glisten of the ocean, its motion, the sky, people and boats, activities of life. She always mentions how much she loves living where she is and how fortunate she is. She voluntarily stopped driving. She walks to her corner grocery store, to the beauty parlor to get her hair done, to the harbor and the beach. Fearful that she will become lost, she always takes the same route. My brother handles the paying of bills. She continues to live successfully by herself.

Where does Rubenfeld Synergy fit into all this? I completed the Rubenfeld Synergy Training two months before Mom's diagnosis. Prior to my entering the training, when Mom would mention her forgetfulness Bill and I would minimize it by saying, "Yeah, that happens to me, too." One moment we'd be trying to convince her how well she was doing; the next we'd become frustrated when she didn't remember something we had just discussed. We had no experience with old people. Our father had died young, our grandparents had died before we'd had a chance to get to know them. And we were in denial.

That soon changed for me. In the Rubenfeld Synergy Training

I discovered that what people want is not my advice—of which I have plenty—but for me to be fully present with them, listen to them, and experience them as they experience themselves. As a result, my hours spent talking with Mom around the kitchen table began to change. Rather than try to deny, minimize, or spin information in a positive way, I was able to hear what she was saying. When we were together I became more interested in her than in myself and I began to ask questions about her childhood. While "Describe your childhood" produced little response, questions such as "What was your favorite room?" and "Who else walked with you to school?" stimulated her memories. As she allowed the memories to surface, I came to see her through her experience.

I wrote a book for her, filled with my memories of events like this one:

> *You are washing dishes looking out the window. You stop, turn, and say, "I just saw two planes collide in midair." We hear it broadcast on the news.*

When Mom read this in the book she said she felt the terror and surprise again, just as she had forty-five years ago. Mom's short-term memory continues to diminish. I can see her listening intently, interested, hearing what I say. Then she tries to recall it and it is gone. She says," I hear it, it comes in, and I'm right there. Then I go to find it and it's gone, as if it went right through me and out a hole in the back of my head."

As she loses her short-term memory, her memories of the deep past seem to be surfacing. For me this brings both discovery and loss. I discover something new about her, a piece of her history or a feeling or thought. When she tells me something new about herself and I discover a piece of her history or a feeling or thought, I am also poignantly aware that there is less of her available for sharing the discovery.

Certain things that I learned and relearned, discovered and explored during the Rubenfeld Synergy Training are gifts that have enriched my life with Mom, both before and since her diagnosis. I don't like that she has Alzheimer's, yet with these gifts I have learned to accept it.

PATIENCE. Ilana often says much of the "magic" of Rubenfeld Synergy is in the w–a–i–t–i–n–g, waiting for tight muscles to release or energy to move. This applies to interactions, too: waiting for Mom to process what I'm asking or to find what she's lost. Or repeating something many times, each time as if it is the first time. I am patient as I guide Mom through Rubenfeld Synergy BodyMind Exercises as she enjoys herself, discovers her own movement, or moves in long-forgotten ways.

Listening to her responses, hearing what she is saying underneath the words, following the metaphors, opening the view to her life. Hearing and seeing her now in reference to her own life instead of in reference to me. Quieting my mind so that I can be with her.

BEING IN THE PRESENT. With Mom I get lots of practice being in the here-and-now, because most moments are new for her even though it may look like repetition to me. Being present with her, keeping my mind quiet and curious and compassionate. When she wants to talk about "how awful it is, losing your mind," about her fear of having a life not worth living, or about her desire for the right to die when she wants to, I can empathize with her and admit I do not have a solution. We are in this together.

HUMOR. I was moved greatly by Deborah Hoffmann's documentary about her own mother's Alzheimer's, *Complaints of a Dutiful Daughter.* As Hoffmann said in an interview, "This is a funny situation. . . . In any other setting, everyone would laugh."

Ilana teaches that humor is healing, that we can travel through the darkest places with the light of laughter. Mom feels safe sharing her feelings, fears, and apprehensions with me, and we laugh a lot. We laugh at stupid things that happen, like using her new microwave. She "just punched the middle three buttons" and after a while it was smoking—those three buttons heated her TV dinner for 45.6 minutes! She surprises herself with her wit and enjoys making us laugh. She does not remember where I park her car, but she recognizes it and remarks on "its cute butt" when we find it.

SELF-CARE. Whenever Mom brought her purse on an outing, the whole trip was about "Where's my purse?" She may well have had it clutched under her arm, or may have left it two stores back. Now I insist that she leave her purse at home. When she asks "Where's my purse?" it's much easier just to say, "You didn't bring it." I do this for my own self-care. Recently she said it is easier for her without her purse; now all she needs to bring is her Kleenex, stuffed in her sleeve. It has become her self-care, too.

RESPECT. Respecting her life; respecting her heart; honoring her as she was then, as she is now, as she will be.

AND CELEBRATION—celebration of my relationship with Mom. It is not the form, it's not the picture, it's not the supposed-to's. It's the acknowledgment of two people meandering through life, wherever that path goes, with whatever equipment and adjustments are required.

Together these gifts have given me the opportunity, self-knowledge, and consequent ability to stand with my mother—to slump with her, cry with her, laugh with her, and walk with her. This is my reward, my gift—to be with her as she is and as I am.

Drawing Upon
EVERYTHING WE ARE

RUBENFELD SYNERGISTS bring to their study and practice a lifetime of experience and wisdom, and their own personal approaches to life. Synergists are encouraged, both in the training and in subsequent ongoing supervision, to make use of every aspect of themselves, in order to inspire clients to do likewise.

The following stories illustrate this richness and diversity in the service of healing. The authors refer to some of their prior or concurrent vocations and avocations: psychotherapist, chiropractor, equestrian, artist, yoga teacher, art therapist, dream analyst. In their work as Synergists they also draw upon experiences that are not reflected in the stories—their years as metalsmith, journalist, administrator, dancer, singer, director, teacher of journaling and meditation, professor of theater arts, practitioner of martial arts.

Practitioners who access all of themselves in their work make it easier for their clients to access all of themselves, too.

Synopses

It Takes More than Talk. After three years of talk therapy, Diane and her client Madelaine* have five months of Rubenfeld Synergy sessions. Diane describes the deepening of Madelaine's work as the two of them bring the wisdom of the body into the experience of therapy.

Feeling the Paint. While on the teaching staff of the current training, Toni, Gay, Donna, and Tanzy describe being coached by Ilana. Gay learns to use her love of painting, and Toni her love of horseback riding, to enhance their "listening hands" and supervisory skills.

Parallel Paths to the Light. Suzanne describes many similarities between Rubenfeld Synergy and the Kripalu Yoga she practiced and taught for many years. Both methods, ancient and modern, helped her and her clients face fear and awaken compassion by tapping into the body's innate, sensate wisdom.

Dreams, My Other Pathway to Healing. Patti describes her self-exploration through dream analysis and the ways in which Rubenfeld Synergy has deepened her ability to understand her dreams and herself.

My Dynamic Duo. Cappi illustrates the synergy between Rubenfeld Synergy and traditional art therapy in a series of sessions with Lisa,* a young anorexic and suicidal client.

The Theatre of Self. Bernard describes his experience of doing a Rubenfeld Synergy demonstration session in front of a group of workshop attendees.

It Takes More
than Talk

Diane Montgomery-Logan

I had been a psychotherapist for several years before Madelaine* came to work with me. She arrived looking for hope after a year of grave despair. A year earlier her husband had betrayed her with behavior she could not bring herself to forgive. By the time she came to see me she had begun to lose her sense of who she was, if not the wife of an honorable man.

Madelaine arrived at my office as I was beginning a three-year training program in the Rubenfeld Synergy Method. During the training I practiced only traditional therapy with Madelaine, relying on language without touch as the primary vehicle for communication. Talk therapy was fairly effective for Madelaine, as it was for many of my clients, but over those three years Madelaine and I came up against its limits. For all the skill she and I both had at using words to access feelings, nonetheless we eventually found ourselves at an impasse: Therapy of the mind and verbal expression of emotions were insufficient for the changes Madelaine wanted to make for herself. Madelaine's story illustrates the dramatic shift that can happen when therapy moves into the non-traditional realm of learning from the body.

During our work in traditional therapy Madelaine labored courageously to come to terms with her past. Despite her physical attractiveness and her loving nature and inquisitive mind, she was self-conscious and retiring, motivated primarily by fear and self-judgment. Her sense of inadequacy showed itself in the way she compared herself to other people. It was there when she limited her choices of career and when she argued with herself as she struggled to leave a husband to whom she was invisible. Her inadequacy was the part of her that selected her clothes and her friends. And it was there in her body when she stood or walked, for she rolled her whole body forward, as though to shrink herself so that no one would see whatever secret she hid. She felt strain in her shoulders and back, as if from the weight of the family messages she had carried for most of her thirty years. Understandably, she was tired.

Madelaine worked hard in therapy. She pounded her rage into many a pillow and wept for all the years without nurturing. She made new friends, took a new job, and shopped for new clothes. But through it all there was a piece missing. Fear was still her primary motivation. In addition, she continued to feel that her husband's choices were in some way her fault. On the deepest levels Madelaine still did not believe she deserved to release herself from her family rules and freely choose her own life. The revolution she had created in her thinking had not filtered down to the deeper levels of her being. There was an essential piece missing in her work of self-transformation.

I recognized this phenomenon, for I had seen it for years with other clients and I had heard other therapists speak of their frustrations as their clients sometimes hit similar impasses. The missing piece was Madelaine's invitation to her body to participate in her therapy. For all her growth in understanding, recognizing, and experiencing her feelings, Madelaine's body still carried the early programming that she was not acceptable. Through three years of therapy Madelaine's nervous system, soft tissues, and skeleton still didn't know that she was entitled to make choices unlike the choices her family had made for generations.

I was caught in an ethical dilemma. During most of these three years I had been practicing Rubenfeld Synergy to help short-term, nonpaying "training" clients move through the same kinds of impasses. And I was increasingly certain this expanded form of therapy was effective. Having been trained as a psychologist, however, I believed that using it with paying clients before I was certified as a Synergist would be unprofessional. So I waited.

Indeed, the shift came for Madelaine when I finished my training and invited her to consider adding the elements of touch and movement to her therapy. Changing from sitting across from me in a chair to lying on a table was a huge shift in our relationship. Her body was rigid as we began that first session. She chose to keep her glasses on and watched me anxiously as I moved around the table, lightly resting my hands on her head or shoulders or hips. Before long, however, her anxiety began to soften as she shifted her attention away from me and toward her inner experience, following it deeply into herself.

As she let down her relentless guard against allowing me to witness her, her muscles and soft tissues began to offer up early family messages for her to reconsider and alter consciously.

Her own words, written between sessions, document this

experience of rediscovering herself. After the first session with touch, she wrote:

> *[I felt] very nervous at first and [had] feelings of being judged and on show. I was anxious that I would get it wrong in some way and that you would finally see the real me. As the session progressed I felt great warmth where you were working. I felt taller afterward! I felt warm, as if I'd just gotten out of a warm bath, relaxed and alert but disoriented, too. It was almost as if I was on a high—like an alcohol buzz. My muscles felt softer, longer. Definitely a sense of strangeness but it wasn't unpleasant. It just felt that I was flowing more naturally—unblocked! Most of all, [I appreciated] the fact that I felt I could control what was happening and that I could say no if I wanted to.*

Madelaine had encountered an experience unlike those she had known in traditional therapy. In all those three years of our sitting across from each other, she had never felt safe enough to relinquish her efforts to project a favorable image to me. Now, in a state of profound awareness, she had allowed herself to be seen fully for one of the few times in her life. She had let her guard down and now she waited.

In the third session, as I touched her left shoulder, she remembered a childhood episode of rejection by her mother. She found herself actively expressing long-denied anger. Afterward she wrote:

> *Very, very powerful—I was shocked by the strength of the emotions I expressed but also pleased (afterward) that I got angry! I defended myself. I felt that I had been through a whirlwind but that I came out stronger, taller, and lighter. I wasn't carrying that pain around anymore.*
>
> *I felt the terror of being abandoned but I wasn't just left*

with it. I moved on to reconnect with my power. The work that you did on my left shoulder while I was lying on my side helped to release all the feelings of fear and clear them out of my system—out of my bones. I also got the chance to revisit that situation and "redo" it—fight back, defend and protect myself. I felt calmer than I had... all week.... I felt very connected to my power and sense of joy and my little child.

Moving her attention from me to herself, Madelaine had freed herself to explore the impact of family relationships and childhood anger on her development. For the first time ever, she had simultaneously experienced and expressed some of her anger and thus had been able to resolve it. Through touch, I had stayed actively present to her without distracting her. What she perceived to be "work that you did on my shoulder" was, in fact, physical and emotional release she herself had done while I was simply touching her shoulder lightly. She had known intuitively how to proceed.

As Madelaine felt increasingly safe with Rubenfeld Synergy, we were gradually able to move our focus to her longing to be authentic with others. After one session, when she felt particularly challenged by my having fully "seen" her, she wrote:

I confronted a lot of feelings of shame and anger about my body—and that I felt used as a child as a weapon in [my] parents' battles. It was terrifying. But this time I had the opportunity to defend myself and fight back. I didn't have that chance as a little girl. My shoulders [became]... looser, more relaxed, softer. A sense of opening up and releasing— instead of my usual pattern of shrinking, closing down. The other feeling, later in the week, was a sense of vulnerability, that I had really been "seen"... a sense that I had unblocked feelings that I had been very ashamed of for a long, long

time....I think that this is an important piece for me. I've
disconnected from and loathed my body for such a long time.
It was good to be able to explore these frightening feelings
and feel safe at the same time.

In this session, instead of talking about and understanding the
"terror of abandonment," Madelaine felt that terror there in the
moment with me. Instead of remembering the choice to hide herself from her mother's seeing her fully and possibly rejecting her,
Madelaine returned to that choice point in the session. Could she
let herself be fully seen by me and thus risk abandonment?
Courageously, she did: Though she had allowed herself to be fully
seen only a few times before, she trusted her body and settled into
the experience with ease.

During the next few months, Madelaine forged a new relationship with her body by reexperiencing on the table both the
negative messages she had received as a girl and her long-buried
anger about them. After one session, in which she revisited her
decision as a young teen to shut down her sexual energy, she wrote:

My relationship to my body has started to change. I notice
that I'm smiling at myself when I look in the mirror now—
instead of grimacing!

[I liked] the chance to expel all those feelings of shame and
self-loathing—to finally be rid of them and to replace those
feelings with a really positive and sensual image of myself. I
am really starting to connect more with my whole body—to
be more appreciative and respectful of it.

In a relatively short time Madelaine had come to a new and unexpectedly friendly relationship with herself as a sensuous, attractive
woman. With subsequent sessions, as Madelaine and I worked to
weave together her reclaimed authenticity and newly discovered

sensuality, she recognized a sense of peace and rightness to her life. Following a session a few weeks later, she wrote:

> *I felt that I really reconnected to a very special place—home. That experience has stayed with me for the remainder of this week. It has been very comforting and wonderful. As if I've reentered a very special place I'd been torn away from years before. The images I visualized during the session were very vivid—almost photographic. I've found that remembering those scenes calms me down and deepens my breathing. It helps to reduce tension throughout my body. The only way I can really describe it is a sense of coming home. To my true home, at last.*
>
> *[I was] putting my feet back on the floor and feeling the solidness and comfort of the floor again! This helped me to really understand that I can bring this experience of God, spirituality, serenity, with me. I didn't have to leave it behind on the table. It took me a while to grasp that the experience of peace was inside me, not external.*

After about five months of Rubenfeld Synergy, Madelaine was offered a job in another part of the country. Though she was reluctant to terminate therapy, we both knew she was prepared to begin the next phase of her life. She had cultivated her ability to attune to her own power and grace. Her body was now her ally in her journey. And now she knew how to decipher the code with which her body spoke to her.

When we said good-bye in the last session, Madelaine wondered if she could find her way without my help. But both of us knew this anxiety was just part of the habitual pattern from her past. Under the anxiety was a rock-solid belief in herself that transcended the doubts and fears her family had taught her. She didn't need to know the details of what life would bring her. It was enough to be ready to welcome it, however it appeared.

Madelaine and I had spent our first three years together trying to gently coax the deeper, symbolic meaning from her story. During that time we had built a sturdy, loving relationship that was the container for Madelaine's deep delving into herself. But it wasn't until we began our work with touch that Madelaine began to literally *embody* her insight and fully integrate into her life the many changes she had made in our earlier therapy. In the five months of our work with Rubenfeld Synergy, Madelaine progressed from understanding that she was entitled to joy to experiencing the richness of claiming her place in life. In those five months she began the journey toward both her softness and her power as a woman.

Feeling the Paint

Toni Luisa Rivera, Gay Marcontell, Donna M. Ulanowski, and P. Tanzy Maxfield

*Toni Luisa (a chiropractor), Gay (an artist),
Donna (a licensed counselor), and Tanzy (a
body-worker and couples therapist) are on
the teaching staff of the current training class.
Here they re-create a supervision session with
Ilana.* —Ed.

TONI LUISA

Ilana asked one of the teaching interns, Donna, to lie on the floor
on her right side with her knees bent, and to demonstrate the
BodyMind Exercise "Sliding Shoulder Blades." This exercise is
ordinarily done by one person alone, but Ilana wanted to use it to
give us ideas for supervising the trainees. In the training week that
was about to start, the trainees would be practicing somatic skills
with clients who are lying on their sides.

First Ilana asked Donna to do the exercise while the other
interns watched. Donna moved her left shoulder slowly up toward
her ear, paused a moment, and then moved it slowly down toward
her hip. Because of my chiropractic training, I got into my usual
discussion with Ilana about what was happening anatomically—

in this case the different muscles that would be used, depending on whether Donna let her elbow bend or kept her elbow straight and let her hand rest on her hip.

Ilana then asked Gay to sit on the floor facing the top of Donna's head and touch Donna's shoulder with "listening hands" while Donna moved it. Then she had Gay move Donna's arm and asked Gay to describe any difference she was aware of in Donna's movement. Gay seemed to be thinking hard and having some difficulty expressing herself. Ilana asked her to "listen" again with her hands to Donna's movement and to try again to speak about it. Gay became frustrated.

Then came the breakthrough. Ilana, who knows that Gay is an artist, asked her to speak about the movement as if she were painting. Gay began to speak of the movements as if they were different brush strokes.

GAY
I need to re-create the scene for myself in order to put it into words.

> I sit on the floor near Donna's head and make myself comfortable so that when I touch her, nothing will impede the flow of information through my body. I bring my hands to join Donna's shoulder during one of the pauses, and, as Donna again moves her shoulder down, I move with it. After I've followed this movement for a while, Ilana asks me to take over the movement *for* Donna.
>
> Ilana asks me to describe what I'm experiencing. I find it difficult to feel and talk at the same time. When it's obvious to everyone that I'm frustrated by the attempt, she encourages me to start over again, this time accessing my visual sense and using the language of art to describe what I am experiencing. At first I continue to struggle to figure

out what she is asking of me. Then I take a breath and just quiet myself into the experience, as if I'm meditating. I am aware of thoughts as they come and go, but I don't feel the need to do anything with them.

Letting go of trying to figure out what I'm supposed to do, I tune in to my hands as they follow Donna's shoulder up and down.

"There is a stroke of paint…," I begin and then stop.

"How big is the stroke?" Ilana urges.

"It is moderately broad, like my thumb from the tip to the first knuckle." I pause as I "watch" Donna's movement with my hands and body and notice slight changes with each repetition of the movement.

"Is there a color?" Ilana prompts.

"The color is a pale reddish orange and the stroke is uneven—heavier, darker, and broader as the movement pauses, then lighter and narrower as the movement speeds up. I see bumps of color within the stroke." I sink deeper into the experience.

"Now it's changing! The stroke is much broader, like my whole thumb from tip to base. The color is more saturated and pure. It sprawls broadly, moving off the one-dimensional surface and coming straight toward me. It is a strong calligraphic stroke."

TONI LUISA

As Gay spoke I could see her going inside and touching a deeper place within herself. She became more intent in her listening and speaking. It was lovely, and as Gay spoke I could observe Donna's movements become smoother and more uniform.

DONNA

I noticed a tremendous change in the quality of Gay's touch. Her hands seemed to come alive. I felt more "received," as if she were actively listening with her whole being, not just her hands. And I felt more listened to throughout *my* whole being, not just in my shoulder. When Gay was focusing on the paint, there was more of a dance, a flow of energy between us. She wasn't just tracking my movement.

Safety is very important to me. After Ilana asked Gay to draw on her artist's sense, and I was to passively let Gay move my shoulder, I felt more trusting than the first time she tried it. I allowed her to move my shoulder more easily.

GAY

This issue of safety is primary when we use touch. "I'm *with* you, not doing something *to* you." I believe the changes I noticed in the stroke and color were due to our nonverbal communication and Donna's level of safety with me, as well as her own interior conversation with herself.

TONI LUISA

What struck me was the paradox—that the more Gay was with Gay and Gay's world of painting, the more she was with Donna and Donna's world of the shoulder movement.

GAY

I felt the change in Donna's muscle tone as she released more into the conversation we were having somatically.

DONNA

You know, when Gay was moving my shoulder I was so deep in that somatic "conversation" that if you had asked me, I might have said it all took place in silence.

GAY

Even though Ilana and I were talking out loud, this coaching session was about nonverbal communication. When we're working with real clients, we can share our images and metaphors with them verbally if it's appropriate. Whether or not we share it, and whether or not they resonate with it, we are all the richer for it because we are richer within ourselves. That day with Ilana, supervision was all about how to use *ourselves*—our lives, our metaphors—to enrich and enliven the somatic connection.

TONI LUISA

Ilana said to Gay, "You should have seen the difference in your face as you contacted that image!" and did a great imitation of the change in Gay's face as she tapped into her artist's sense. I noticed the way Gay's voice and energy became softer as she spoke, and Donna's movements became smoother and more flowing.

Then I asked Ilana, "This approach is all well and good for someone who has a metaphor like painting to use, but what am I to use? My mind always goes to the intellectual: I visualize the bones and muscles that are moving, or I identify adhesions. Everything is very concrete and anatomical."

In response Ilana invited me to work with Tanzy's shoulder. When I was positioned at Tanzy's head, Ilana asked me what *I* most liked to do. Being a horsewoman I said, "Riding." She asked me to move Tanzy's shoulder and use riding as the metaphor. I did so and, when I noticed a slight glitch in the movement, my mind jumped to the transitions in riding, where the goal is to have the transitions—from walk to trot, from canter to walk—be as smooth as possible.

As I spoke of this out loud, Tanzy's arm began to make the transition from the upward movement to the downward movement and vice versa in a much smoother way. I was so involved in what I was saying that I didn't pay much attention at all to Tanzy or her shoulder. She seemed to fade into the background, though of course I did notice the change in the quality of the movement.

TANZY

While Toni Luisa was telling Ilana about the transitions in riding, I felt that she was much more present with me than before, and I, too, noticed my shoulder movements getting smoother in response to their conversation about riding.

GAY

It is interesting how everyone remembers this session differently. We have access only to our own experience. To get another's we have to ask.

DONNA

This coaching session dramatically illustrated a truth that I have learned and relearned countless times in my training and practice: Only when we are fully in touch with our whole selves can we be fully in touch with our clients. And only then can they become fully in touch with themselves.

Parallel Paths to the Light

Suzanne Selby Grenager

In the early seventies my dearest childhood friend, Lucy, began a hideous, heartrending battle with cancer, at the age of twenty-eight. I'd been following her slow decline closely, by phone, letter, and visits whenever possible. No one, including her husband, a physician, ever said Lucy was dying. Still, about a week before she died, I sensed it was time to be with her again. I packed a small bag, left my husband, young child, and job, and caught a train to New York.

It had been less than two months since I'd last seen Lucy. But for one sickening moment I did not recognize the bald, ruined skeleton of a woman the nurse wheeled out, with a breezy, "Here she is." I was shocked beyond words, and ashamed not to have known my friend. So began the most grueling week of my life.

To my surprise this painful bedside vigil became the spark for my spiritual birth. Watching Lucy go so finally to sleep served to wake me up. After thirty years of hiding out in my head, I started coming alive in my skin. But the process of getting to know and accept myself—body, mind, and emotions—proved exceedingly difficult. In the six months following Lucy's death, the lid to Pandora's box flew off, revealing a lifetime's stash of horrific psychic pain—fear, grief, anger, and shame. I was besieged by nightmares, insomnia, chest pains, and—once, after taking only half a low-dose Valium prescribed by my doctor—hallucinations. Terrified, I thought I, too, was about to die.

Fortunately help was on the horizon, in the form of two seemingly different but remarkably parallel paths to the light. Over the next several years, a three-thousand-year-old Eastern spiritual tradition and a contemporary Western therapy helped me understand that in order to break through fear and reach love, I would have to reinhabit my body, temple of the spirit we all essentially are. I was very fortunate that both Kripalu Yoga and Rubenfeld Synergy offer practical, *body*-based tools to help me—and later, hundreds of students and clients—get out of our minds, tap into our bodies' innate, sensate wisdom, and experience love.

The first leg of my odyssey took me to Kripalu Yoga, a spiritually rich mix of traditional Hatha and Bhakti Yogas (the paths of right action and devotion, respectively), designed for Americans by a charismatic teacher. For the next fifteen years Kripalu—the Center, its guru, and staff as well as the yoga itself—offered me what amounted to a master's degree in conscious, compassionate living. At Kripalu and at home alone on the floor, I learned to use yoga postures, breathing, meditation, and devotional techniques to relax deep into my being and to trust what I felt.

Spurred by my need for emotional healing, I gradually re-created my personal yoga practice as a kind of psychotherapy-in-motion.[1] Instead of following a standard sequence of *asanas*,[2] I'd lie on the floor, relax, breathe, and tune in to the knot in my throat or the ache in my shoulder. I'd wait, I'd see, I'd feel whatever was most alive in me.

As I lay waiting and feeling, I'd notice physical urges to move in this way or that. When I chose to follow them, I'd often be guided naturally into positions that let me more fully feel and attend to my pain. I'd pay extra attention whenever I sensed emotion lurking around a physical discomfort, and I'd make small, exploratory movements to heighten my awareness—a hallmark of the Kripalu approach (and, as I later discovered, of the Rubenfeld Synergy Method as well). In order to release all the tension I could, I made a lot of noise—sighing, grunting, laughing, crying, sometimes coughing until I almost choked.

I'd regularly be drawn into some awkward-looking variation of the shoulder stand pose. Taking long, deep breaths and trying not to control my body with my mind, I'd find myself softening into the same uncomfortable physical sensations that I usually sought to avoid. I'd continue gently holding the posture as long as I could. When I was lucky, my locked shoulders and tight chest would begin to let go.

With energy streaming from my sore, tight muscles and nerves, I would sometimes shake uncontrollably. Especially in the shoulder stand, which compresses and then releases the chest and throat, I often ended up wailing like a forlorn child. "Mommy, where are you?" I would cry. "Why don't you love me? I need you to love me." Although surprised by these outbursts at first, I remembered it's the chest that houses the heart—and the throat, the voice. By stimulating both, I was able finally to give deep, old feelings their voice.

---

[1] This was in the days before yoga therapies had been developed.

[2] The Sanskrit word for yoga postures.

My mother did her best but, since *her* mother was as cold as ice, Mom knew next to nothing about the unconditional love for which I had longed as a child. Thanks to my customized yoga practice, though, the adult I had become was finally making time and space for "Little Suzie." As I allowed the child I once was to feel *her* pain, I experienced compassion for myself—then and now. "Poor Suzie," I would find myself moaning, after my tears were spent. "I'm sorry you're hurting. You're a good girl.... I love you." And so I did, at least for a few precious minutes, as I'd rest with my arms wrapped around myself.

By the late eighties, however, my practice of yoga-as-therapy had stalled. I had begun to experience some frightening bouts of what felt like shame. Like an itch I couldn't quite reach, it eluded my efforts to get to the bottom of it through yoga alone. Because several long-term yoga students also seemed ready to delve deeper than I could take them in class, my teaching, too, was less satisfying than before.

My frustration peaked the summer Ilana Rubenfeld came to town. I attended her weeklong workshop and watched as one demonstration client after another tackled tough emotions in much the way I'd been wanting my students to do. Before the week was out I'd committed to a long, costly training program in far-off, frigid Toronto.

Although I'm not now practicing Rubenfeld Synergy, I consider the time and money well spent. The training experience, coupled with required private sessions back home, helped me pick up my emotional clearing work where I'd left off with yoga. Immediately the shame I'd been sensing intensified. I found myself reexperiencing my deepest childhood fear—of daring to be myself with people I saw as powerful.

In Toronto, for one intense week at a time, I was faced with a charismatic and authoritative master teacher who reminded me of my lovely but demanding mother. "Why can't you be just like me, dear?" was the message Little Suzie had gathered from Mom. Now Big Suzie, who was still ashamed of not being enough like her mother, felt she was getting this message again—from the teacher and, by extension, her staff.

As their student I found myself seeking their approval as desperately as I had once sought Mother's love. At the same time, I felt totally—if irrationally—incapable of measuring up. In this psychic re-creation of my family scenario I was so busy putting on masks, in order to conform and "get it right," that when I did get approval I felt it was for these false selves. Little got through to the "real me." I felt intimidated, vulnerable, and at times so ashamed that I almost quit.

Somehow, though, I stuck it out. Thanks to the depth of the Rubenfeld work and the sheer length of the training, the pain of keeping myself down finally got harder to bear than the fear of having an unlovable self show up and be judged as unacceptably different. Toward the end, exhausted from both mask making and mining all that shame, forty-some years of defenses fell and I began to emerge from my shell.

Much as in the aftermath of Lucy's death, it was my willingness to be *in* extreme emotional turmoil that got me *out* of it. Both times the pain was so great that I needed more encouragement than I knew how to give myself.

Although Rubenfeld Synergy works with feelings more explicitly and, I believe, more effectively than does classical yoga, the two disciplines have much in common: Both invite us to set aside the mind and its conditioned thoughts, and to pay attention to the body. For, unlike the mind, the body doesn't lie. Both systems promote trust in our physical inclinations by having us lie down, relax, breathe with awareness, and explore sensations with gentle movements. What's more, both approaches recognize that the body can be a gateway to transcendence: in yoga through meditation; in Rubenfeld Synergy through a trance-like state of deep, intuitive relaxation.

Most critically, perhaps, both systems understand that before we can *trans*cend, we must *des*cend, to clear pain both physical and psychic. And in order to let feelings go, we must first let them come and be felt fully in the body. The teachings (and, up to a point, my practice) of Kripalu Yoga taught me two related lessons: First, that troubling emotions will live in us and fester until we feel, express, and release them, or until we integrate them into our being. Second, that the moment we succeed in letting go of our fear, anger, grief, and shame—by whatever means—the kinder, gentler states of joy, peace, compassion, and love are right there, available to nourish us.

To illustrate how well the troubled body can serve as a gateway to repressed feelings, and, by clearing them, to the compassionate (or so-called "higher") self, I'd like to recall a Rubenfeld Synergy session with a client I'll call Diane.*

Diane is a strong, down-to-earth woman I first knew as my yoga student. She climbs onto the table and lies belly-up. This position, with back to the Earth, is much like the classic yoga relaxation pose, *savasana* ("the corpse"). It sharpens the senses and creates more space for the heart, lungs, and guts, while letting the mind settle into the body. I begin by lightly touching Diane's head and then move to her feet, reassuring her wordlessly, "I'm here with you on your terms; you are safe in my hands." I notice at once that her ankles feel rigid, suggesting that her legs and hips might be tight.

As I walk slowly back to the head of the table, I hear

Diane's strangely uneven breath—an indication, I know from both yoga and my Rubenfeld training, that her "life force" is somehow awry. So I am careful to approach her head in slow motion before I cup it in my hands and gently roll it from side to side. Diane holds on at the neck, too, resisting my hands in a way she usually does not.

Though Diane is a person who volunteers little, she responds well to the slightest prompting. So I ask simply, "What's going on here?" while using my hands to exchange informative energy with her right leg and hip.

She answers that a long-standing hip pain has become chronic and now hurts so much she nearly canceled our appointment. As I carefully lift and hold her leg in my arms, the tension in the hip is palpable. I sense that we are on to a possible window into a psychic pain behind the physical one. With words, touch, and gentle movement I subtly encourage Diane to keep her attention on her hip (to "hold the posture," as we say in yoga).

"Can you tell me how it feels?" I ask, as I continue to cradle her right leg and move it slowly in all directions.

When Diane says how much it hurts and how tired she is of having to deal with this "damned hip," I suggest that she tune in further and direct her relaxed, receptive awareness into the sore hip. As I continue holding and rocking her leg like a baby, I feel her let go a little, which makes me—and, I suspect, her—all the more conscious of how tightly she is still holding on.

Diane remains quiet, even as she begins to look distraught. I ask if there's anything she wants to "say" to her hip or that her hip might want to say to her. Without hesitation she blurts out, "It's not fair." Then, more upset still,

"I didn't do anything to deserve this!"

I gently lower her leg and place my hands underneath the sore hip to support it. I feel a torrent of energy, like a blast of warm air. Sensing a reservoir of fear and possibly anger, I invite Diane to repeat what she just said for as long as she wants. I suggest she follow her words wherever they lead her that she is willing to go.

Diane takes to this idea at once. "It's not fair!" she bellows. "I don't deserve this!" As her outrage escalates, her face starts to contort, and she wriggles her hands and body this way and that as if to escape from some demon I can't see. I've never known this self-contained woman to be so wrought up.

"I don't deserve this!" she wails again, like a distraught child. I urge her to stay with it. I know that "holding the verbal and emotional posture," in this Rubenfeld Synergy counterpart to the physical holding in yoga, may allow Diane to unearth any emotional hurt beneath her pain. Finally I sense a shift, as if Diane's scattered energy has found a focus. "Where are you right now?" I ask.

Without hesitation Diane begins to describe the street she walked every day from home to school when she was six. She tells me, as if it were happening as she speaks, that she is walking by herself one morning, when a strange car pulls over to the curb. The driver stops his car and calls out the window for directions. As she approaches the car, he opens the door and exposes himself to her. After a moment he slams the door and speeds off.

As Diane describes this experience from start to finish, she seems to be not so much retelling it as reliving it. Her expressions shift dramatically from moment to moment and her hands twist and clench as, she later told me, they used to do when she'd get upset as a kid. And she has turned over onto her side, drawing her legs up into the fetal position as if to protect herself.

Knowing that what we resist persists, I encourage Diane to really let the experience in and even, at the appropriate point, to look with her mind's eye right at the man's exposed member. She does, and this time, instead of clamming up and shutting down in shame, she becomes furious and starts to tell the "jerk" just what she thinks of him. Through tumultuous tears she boldly expresses the fear and outrage the six-year-old could not—feelings that have been bottled up for thirty years as shame. When she is spent from crying and ranting, Diane sinks easily into a soft clarity and calm. Quietly she speaks words of comfort and forgiveness to her "little girl" while gently patting and rocking herself. At the end of the session, Diane is exhausted but radiant.

Later she wrote to me about her experience of the session.

In my many attempts over the years to face and release that painful incident, this was the first time I fully felt again like a six-year-old, confused, ashamed and angry. . . . At last I saw and knew that the little girl I had been was totally innocent. I had done nothing. I was not wrong or stupid. I finally understood and believed that this terrible experience I had held myself accountable for over the years was in no way my fault. Now, instead of assuming I should have done something to avoid the man, as I always had, I was absolutely clear that to handle the situation any differently was way beyond the experience of the beloved and petted baby of the family I was at six. My little girl had never known anything but good from grown men and could only have expected that.

About her hip pain Diane wrote, "When I got off the table, I was comfortable. I drove home with little pain and have been more hopeful of a complete recovery ever since."

Although Diane's healing was unusually dramatic, I was consistently delighted by the power of Rubenfeld Synergy to heal and awaken even clients who lacked Diane's spiritual preparation through yoga. For example, three different women with no such training inadvertently tapped into the universal energy or "life force" that yogis refer to as *prana,* the Chinese as *chi,* and we in the West as "spirit."

Shortly after lying down and closing her eyes, each woman found a part of her body beginning to move on its own. As she became absorbed in her particular "meditation in motion" (as we called this fairly common phenomenon at Kripalu), each was able to "give voice" to the upstart arm or foot and learn something important that it had to "tell" her about a troublesome, unresolved problem with another person. These sessions, like Diane's, ended with the clients feeling understanding and compassion, for themselves, at least.

I am always inspired by such moments of "transcendent" experience, in which the human spirit is made manifest. I relish the tangible, audible proof they offer that we mortals are more than our aging bodies, madcap minds, and bewildering emotions.

I am grateful that, thanks to Kripalu Yoga and the Rubenfeld Synergy Method, I have had many chances to come face to face with our marvelous human capacity to transcend, to trust, and to express the love that is our essence. Most of all, I am touched that it was through losing my best friend that I began to find that essence in myself, and that my heart-opening journey began—ironically—on Valentine's Day, the day that Lucy died.

Dreams, My Other Pathway to Healing

Patti Allen

I was always a dreamer, but not in the sense of having unrealistic or unattainable daydreams. No, I was a nocturnal dreamer, one who dreamed frequently and remembered seldom. Most of my dream images would quickly evaporate in the light of day. Once in a while, though, one would stay with me, shadowing my day and tracking my every move, as if to say, "Look at me! I am important." When finally a dream challenged me enough to remember it, I surrendered and wrote it down, thinking about it as if it were a riddle to unravel or a puzzle to solve.

Nine months before I began the Rubenfeld Synergy Training Program, I wrote in my journal:

*I've denied so much of myself over the years that I doubt that
I'd allow myself to recognize whatever might present itself
[as the path to follow]. So I think I'll try this Rubenfeld
thing...shake myself up...do something new. One thing
may lead to another.*

I went to bed after writing that and had a flying dream. Two other
people flew with me. I wondered who they might be.

At the time, I felt that dreams were safe to explore. All my life
I had kept my feelings buried deep below the surface. Exploring
dreams allowed me to remain detached and not have to take them
personally. In the way that a dream involves other people, and in
its non-reality or other-worldliness while retaining a storylike
quality, I found exploring one as safe as discussing a mystery
novel. In time I became the tracker, hot on the trail of my inner
self. I came to see each dream as a fragment of my unconscious, a
fragment that might give me a fuller, multidimensional understanding of my Self.

And so I began my training in December 1991 in this fertile
dream soil that I had barely begun to till. As part of the three-year
training, we were required to have a minimum of twenty private
Rubenfeld Synergy sessions per year. These sessions took me
beyond the intellectual interpretation of my dreams and added to
my awareness the physical and emotional dimensions that had
been lacking. After finishing my first training week in New York,
I had this dream:

*I have just given birth to a baby boy. I am the surrogate for
a woman I know who looks pregnant but that's only for
"show." Before I can give the baby to her, the baby starts to
move and communicate in ways that are incredible for a
newborn. I call her husband over to show him, but he can't*

see anything out of the ordinary. I tell him that just because he doesn't see it or acknowledge it, doesn't mean it isn't so.... This baby is becoming an amazing genius and a freak monster. I am in awe and repelled at the same time.

In a session after I had this dream, my Rubenfeld Synergist asked me what part of the dream had the most energy for me or most interested me. We then explored what it was like to be pregnant, to be full and round with life—a life that belonged to someone else! What was it like to give that life away and where did I feel that in my body? The key to this dream was my awareness that I felt this pregnancy not in my belly, as one might imagine, but in my heart. It felt as if a chunk of my heart were being taken out and given away, piece by piece, bit by bit, and all with my help! With this new insight, originating in my body, my energy shifted and my shoulders began to relax into the table.

We continued to explore my body's reactions to seeing the baby move and talk in ways that newborns don't normally talk. I discovered that feeling awed and repelled at the same time was echoed in my feet! My right foot pointed in one direction, my left foot in the other. The left was heavier, more in contact with the table than the right. My left foot recoiled from that baby; the right foot moved forward, toward the baby. And when your own two feet want to move in two different directions, the results are immobilization—or, as I sometimes call it, "the fine art of staying stuck!" As soon as I experienced my feet as feeling stuck, my immediate reaction was to move them. I saw my feet's stuckness as a metaphor for my life and, with this new awareness, I began to integrate the information into my whole being. Focusing on how I felt, in the present, about the images in the dream was very different from just thinking about them.

Through my Synergist's use of touch and her focus on my

awareness of my body, my feelings slowly began to emerge from the dreamwork. Paradoxically my feelings, which I had for so long tried to keep out of my awareness, proved to be the key to understanding my dreams and myself. I could no longer ignore my feelings and keep them at arm's length. They turned out to be less frightening than I had feared because my body was engaged in the process and kept me grounded. Being grounded meant focusing on the "here and now," on what is, rather than on what might or might not happen in the future. In a session I could feel my solidity and strength. I felt like a tree, with my roots reaching deep into the earth, keeping me upright, even when the emotional winds blew. Or in the words of one of my clients, with whom I have since done dreamwork, "I wasn't alone. I had my body."

During the three-year period of my training, I recorded over one hundred dreams in my journal. I returned to and reviewed this written record so many times that it became my "State of the Union" address—the "union" of my unconscious and conscious selves. These dreams provided me with insights and awareness that my conscious, waking self either had no knowledge of or viewed in a different way. The journal allowed me to recognize patterns of dreams with symbols, images, and themes in common, patterns that I would have missed had I not written them down. Common dream symbols during this time of change and self-discovery included babies and births, California (the place of my childhood), earthquakes and fires, mud and water, dark men giving chase, storms in the distance, speeding cars, and wild animals and insects of all kinds. These dreams were my signposts and barometers.

I dreamed:

We are back at our old house in California. I look in the garage, at what I think is my car, and I realize that isn't my license plate. Then, looking closer, I realize that isn't my car, either! Suddenly, there is an earthquake. It is quite strong and the shaking goes on for a while. When it is over I have a definite sense of "That wasn't so bad—I survived!" I awake feeling I could survive any "shake-up."

In session:

My mind still remains part of the process, only now it's not the only process. I understand that the setting of this dream is in my childhood, and the car (my life) that I'm driving (living) isn't my own. This much I would have understood without Rubenfeld Synergy. Adding my body awareness to the equation, I feel the earthquake inside of me, as energy streams through me, giving me a visceral sense of surviving any shake-up of my psyche.

When I think back to that initial journal entry where I wrote "I'll shake myself up," the saying "Be careful what you wish for…" comes to mind!

During my training to become a Synergist, I was ambivalent about taking my turn as a client in one of Ilana's demos. Feeling vulnerable, I hesitated. "Should I? Shouldn't I?" I decided to leave it up to my unconscious: If I had a dream that I remembered, I would get on the table. Sure enough, I had one. In this dream what stood out for me was the image of a broken red candle, which I was rushing to clean up before company arrived.

The next day I volunteered. In the session, Ilana invited me to "become" the candle and describe myself as the candle. "I'm red and I am broken in many pieces." The session took off from there and, as my body began to shake, I could feel the accuracy of my dream image.

I recently watched the videotape of that session and was struck by several points that Ilana made during the group discussion that followed the session, points that I believe to be important to our work as Rubenfeld Synergists, whether or not we are working with dreams. She enjoined us to place no judgments on the form or quality of our clients' process of catharsis. Some people release feelings and emotions with buckets of tears; others may shed a single tear or even none. The single tear I had shed in my session wasn't any less powerful, she said, than were other people's buckets of tears.

Ilana also said that my session might have appeared on the surface as if "not much was happening," but actually it was an example of a client doing work on a very deep level in what some would call an altered state. She also pointed out that to hurry my process along in any way, in order to make it appear that something was happening, would have been to disregard my individual pace and needs as a client. Being rushed was the very situation my unconscious had presented to me in my dream, and therefore, quite possibly, was a common situation for me. As Synergist Ilana had wanted to support me in finding my own pace, and that is in fact what she facilitated in the session. I was allowed the experience of doing the session in my own time and my own way. At the end of the discussion, I named the session *I'll Light My Candle When I'm Ready.*

After my certification as a Rubenfeld Synergist, I continued to study and learn about dreams. Academically I read any book on dreams I could get my hands on, while personally I kept dreaming. The more dramatic images and symbols became less dramatic and less frightening. In their place new symbols and images continued to shake me up in new ways! That's what dreams do. They tell us to "Wake up and pay attention!" As my dreams continued to evolve, I began to find treasures buried in the dirt, and my grandmother's trinkets (another dream image) became my jewels. When I needed help with a decision, I slept on it.

I dreamed:

> *There is a performer, a combination of Joan Rivers and Judy
> Garland, who is rehearsing onstage for an upcoming show in
> an open amphitheater that feels like Vegas. I am there on-
> stage with her and treated as an honored visitor. I don't
> understand, in the dream, why I am there or why I am hon-
> ored. The star asks me to do something like sing or dance and
> I'm confused and embarrassed, not sure what she wants or
> that I can do it. I see a crow fly by. I tell her that's a good
> omen. It seems that being able to read the omen gets me off
> the hook in some way.... [There is] something about the song
> "Somewhere Over the Rainbow." Am I supposed to sing it?
> I explain [to her] that it is a song expressing hope.*

If I'm not yet completely ready to reintegrate my "star" part, I am
willing to be on the stage and "read the omens." Toward that end,
I began teaching others how to work with their dreams and doing
lectures on self-understanding through dreamwork. Because I am
a Rubenfeld Synergist, helping my clients look inside themselves
requires my looking inside myself. My dreams continue to be my
internal roadmap for this process.

Oh, and that flying dream I had after deciding to become a
Rubenfeld Synergist? I can now imagine, though I don't actually
remember, who the two others were who flew with me. On a
metaphorical level they are dreams on one side and the Rubenfeld
Synergy Method on the other. But on a physical reality level, on
the "I can read the omens" level, the two who flew with me are my
Rubenfeld Synergy teachers, who supported me in my personal
growth and dream exploration during my training. I love it when
the various elements of a dream all fall into place. In this dream
the Rubenfeld Synergy Method and dreamwork have been my
pathways to healing and it has all fallen into place.

My Dynamic Duo:

RUBENFELD SYNERGY AND ART THERAPY

Margaret Cappi Lang

It is 1991. I am sitting at the charting desk at St. Luke's Hospital in Phoenix, Arizona, updating my patients' charts with notes about our most recent therapy sessions. For some time I have felt that these patients in the hospital's eating disorder program need something beyond traditional psychotherapy, something even beyond the creative arts therapy that I do with them.

As I chart I think of Elaine Rapp, one of my teachers at Pratt Institute, where I studied art therapy. Elaine had studied with Alexander Lowen, a student of Wilhelm Reich, both of whom were pioneers in working with the body to release old emotional wounds and allow healing to occur. I remember the bodywork that Elaine did with us. I was so impressed with it at the time that I asked her how I could learn to do it. She responded that when the time was right I would find a teacher.

As I recall Elaine's answer I silently ask, "Where are you, teacher?" At that moment a secretary who is walking by accidentally drops a flyer right onto the chart I am working on. I pick up the flyer and read about a workshop being given in Scottsdale, Arizona, by Ilana Rubenfeld, the founder of the Rubenfeld Synergy Method. I finish my charting and take the flyer with me to the art room. While the patients are creating their artwork, I fill out the registration form. I have made my decision without a second thought. I have a sense of knowing!

I am at the workshop. Ilana is demonstrating the work with a volunteer. I feel energy flow through me. I know! I know I am going to learn this powerful work. I know it will help my most difficult and wounded patients. I know! This moment begins an incredible adventure and journey into my own healing and that of my patients, as well. I sign up for the Rubenfeld Synergy Training and start on the adventure of my life. It is a small part of this adventure and journey that I wish to share here, a story of my work with one client.

> *I first met Lisa* in the hospital's art room in 1986, when she was twenty-five. She was late for our first appointment. She had jumped ship and broken the program's "no exercise" rule by going Rollerblading. After a nurse retrieved her, Lisa skated in, a skeleton on wheels with a mischievous grin on her face, defiant. Anorexic and bulimic since she was sixteen, she was in the hospital after a suicide attempt. I also knew that she had been shoplifting for several years, yet I liked her pluckiness, her tenacity. We did art therapy together for several months after this, and she healed parts of herself.*

In 1992 Lisa re-appears, still a skeleton and again suicidal. This time we meet in my studio-office. Her psychotherapist has heard of my work—combining art therapy with Rubenfeld Synergy—and has suggested that Lisa try it. Each of our sessions follows the same pattern: a Rubenfeld Synergy session with Lisa on the table, followed by Lisa's drawing a picture.

In Lisa's first session, as I touch her I notice that her body is extremely tight, both to the eye and to the touch. She flinches when I touch her foot. I decide to introduce touch gradually over the next few sessions, to start by touching only her head and shoulders. After the Rubenfeld Synergy session on the table, Lisa makes a drawing. The drawing, a huge black cloud, communicates the scope of her depression. To my trained art therapist's eye, there are also indications of anxiety and a wish to cover up and hide her pelvic area.

In her second session Lisa chooses to work lying on her side. I cradle her head with one hand and put my other hand on her back and shoulder. She describes three parts of herself: four-year-old Sara, who is scared and helpless as she is picked on by her brothers; six-year-old Tomboy, who is tough, can take care of "himself" and steals; and Amelia, the helpless adult who tries to deal with Sara and Tomboy. The drawing she makes this time depicts the three aspects of herself that she described. In the drawing none of the figures has a body below the waist. I see this as another indication of her depression and anger.

In session three Lisa says she is afraid of my touch. She lies on her side, curled up, and we talk. I stay close but do not touch her. She says she wants nurturing but does not deserve it because she steals. Lisa describes a cycle of wanting nurturing, being denied nurturing, becoming angry and stealing, and then punishing herself by denying herself food and companionship.

Lisa brings a drawing to her fourth session. It depicts adults fighting and a scared child cowering in the corner. These images are disturbing. She curls up on the table and describes her feelings of despair and pain. She talks about how her brothers called her ugly and teased her relentlessly. She feels helpless. With her permission I place one hand gently on her back, the other on her head. She reaches out to me. I take her hand and hold it. I feel her body release some tension and soften a bit. She says, of the drawing she makes afterwards, that it depicts the death of her soul, the loss of her power.

In the fifth session Lisa lies on the table and says she is a big baby, afraid of touch, afraid of life. She reaches her hands up toward me. I take them in mine. She grabs me harder and then releases her grasp, saying she is afraid she will grab on too hard and frighten me, use me up. I say I will tell her if it is too hard. I take her hands. She holds on. She scarcely breathes. I rest my hand lightly over her heart. She says my hand weighs a ton. Her body energy communicates to me a feeling of heaviness and tension around the chest, lungs, and heart. The story of her brothers sitting on her chest emerges. She can't breathe or speak. She is desperate. She holds on to my hands. After a while she says she has gotten in touch with a little part of her heart that can feel. She draws a picture of her heart and the part of it she has reclaimed. I believe this is the beginning of a breakthrough for Lisa.

In the next several sessions Lisa becomes more aware of feelings in her body, especially feelings of holding on in her shoulders and anus. Her hips are loose; her anus holds and controls. In one session she notices anger and releases some of it. After the release she senses blackness. She allows me to touch and work with her shoulders. In another session she clutches my hands from time to time and tells me that she is afraid that I will leave her. She remembers her mother complaining that Lisa "cost too much." Lisa asks me not to leave her. I say, "I am not going anywhere." Her body relaxes and then stiffens again into a rod. She relaxes again and asks to be held. As I hold her, I feel her body soften and release its tension. She says the black cloud is breaking up. One of her drawings shows the cloud becoming less dense. Lisa uses more colors in these drawings, and they have more space and movement than earlier drawings.

At one point during our work together, before I go away on a trip, Lisa expresses concern that I might die on the plane. She asks me to work with her feet and then her head. She reaches for my hand as I do a "head roll," placing my palm on her forehead and gently rolling her head from side to side. I take her hand and place it under mine on her forehead. Together, we roll her head. I see her breathe more deeply and relax. I take away my hand and she continues to roll her head by herself. This movement seems to comfort her; she feels calmer and her body releases some more tension. She says that she can move her own head and asks to borrow one of my stuffed bears while I'm away. Her drawing shows me holding her down by her ankles, grounding her and keeping her from drifting off the Earth into the black cloud of depression.

As time goes on Lisa becomes frightened again. Her drawings depict her shattered in many pieces. Once, she asks me to cover her with a blanket and hold her hand. As I stroke her back and shoulders, she asks me to sing her a song. Sensing her fear, I sing the lullaby "Lavender Blue, Dilly Dilly." Later, her drawing shows me sweeping her up, with the fragments of herself beginning to take form.

In subsequent sessions Lisa begins to feel something other than depression—an energy, a more positive energy. She now allows me to work with her feet and hips as well as her head and shoulders. Her body is relaxed most of the time, becoming stiff and rigid only occasionally. Lisa says she is in touch with someone yelling in her head, saying, "Get it out, just tell." In a session in which Lisa describes herself as a shattered vase, she draws a shattered vase that has a base, a foundation on which Lisa can now build. She says that our work together is helping her to glue her vase back together and that "this is powerful work."

As we continue working together, Lisa gradually develops a playfulness. During one of these playful periods "Sara" and "Tomboy" do a drawing together of fruit—"the fruits of my labor," Lisa says, laughing. She smells the scented markers and laughs again. Lisa comes in after this fruit-drawing session and suggests that we each write a story about our work together. We do so.

My Story

Once upon a time there was a family where a small child was traumatized by the father and brothers. The parents fought, the brothers fought. The mother used the child for her own nurturance after her first husband, a raging alcoholic, left and her second husband, an abuser, died. The mother was so drained by supporting the family—and having been abused herself—that she was empty and had nothing to give the child. She became angry at the little girl, whom she experienced as wanting too much and never being satisfied. She said "grow up" and "quit sniffling."

When the mother went to work, the brothers wrestled with her and teased and molested the little girl. She fought back and acted tough when they called her "baby" and "brat." She tried to call her mother for help, but they prevented her. She raged and was hurt more. So she retreated to the corner, where she was afraid to move, to make a sound, or even to breathe. She lost hope and was shattered. However, inside her was a strength, a light, a heart that she experienced from time to time. She reached toward the light and the heart with all her strength and tried to pull them toward her. Something pulled against her, but she did not give up. She kept on reaching and pulling. She sensed her good mind and her strong legs. In her torso, though, she felt an emptiness. A voice called out to her, "Tell."

With gentle touch, awareness, experimentation, and love, she begins to tell me her story and to put together her shattered self, to integrate her shattered parts. She reaches out. I take her hand. I remain present and patient. We play together. She learns to touch, nurture and hold herself.

Lisa's Story

This has been an emotional journey that has oftentimes been unpleasant; a process of unlocking various doors that emit only glimpses of light, often in cryptic form. When the information revealed is overwhelming, the defensive parts of me slam the doors shut, out of fear. The Rubenfeld Synergy, art therapy, dreamwork, and analysis of transference issues have deciphered the messages. Yet this is a painstaking process that one would easily give up if there were not a companion/witness/guide/safety net to accompany one along the path.

Because my body has so much protective armor, I was not even aware of the many emotions buried beneath the skin until the Rubenfeld Synergy facilitated their release. Cappi's gentle touch evoked sadness and longing for the nurturing lacking in my childhood, along with terror that she might hurt me with that same physical contact. However, because she did not touch beyond my comfort level at various stages of the process, I was able to slowly develop trust that provided me the safety in which to experience the terror, express the anger, and accept the comforting she offered. The Rubenfeld Synergy evoked images that I was unable to access previously via hypnosis alone. Also, it gave permission to the various aspects within me to dialogue with each other so they now understand each other better and, therefore, eventually, may be able to interact more harmoniously.

The art therapy, which included symbols from dreams, served to bypass my intellectualization. The symbols gave Cappi information that I could not put into words because, once again, I was not even aware of the information regarding early trauma that was stored within me at a preverbal level. In addition, the artwork was visual evidence of aspects of my life that I could not rationalize away as easily as I did with straight "talk" therapy.

Finally, the permissiveness and genuine concern that both processes encompass allowed me to express my feelings toward Cappi without fear of judgment, abandonment, or retaliation. This provided a corrective parenting experience. I now understand those were transference feelings I could not safely express in my family of origin. The journey continues as the enigma of the past slowly unfolds in treatment with someone who will hold my hand for support and clarification as we move toward the light of healing.

LISA AND I wrote these stories three years ago. Today Lisa is the mother of a six-month-old baby. She is doing well in her chosen field and in a relationship that promises to be a healthy one. She still struggles with her eating disorder but seems to have the upper hand.

I continue to use my "dynamic duo"—Rubenfeld Synergy and art therapy—with my clients. These two therapies have come together as partners in a dance, weaving their threads together to produce healing, growth, positive changes, and artistry. I am grateful and appreciative of this work, which touches and reveals the soul.

The Theatre of Self

Bernard Coyne

Bernard often draws on his forty years' experience in the theater when he presents Rubenfeld Synergy at large conferences. Here he expresses poetically his personal experience of these presentations.—Ed.

I say, "Who would like to experience Rubenfeld Synergy?" What will happen? I never know as I stand here in front of this conference, this large group of people, like a priest-shaman of old. I am in wonder of "the now" and in the wonder that connects me to ancient campfires and the people who came from all over Greece on the festival of Dionysus to see the gods act out their stories.

This is an experience of the first time. There is a wave of energy in the crowd. Who will be the chosen one? Hands dart up. The woman in the third row has the energy. I invite her and she begins to walk the firewalk of faith, from the community circle to the center. She is the one who makes this act sacred; she represents all of us. The heroine's journey has begun. Everything is heightened. There is a rich silence. Time stands still. This is true theatre, where the divine in the person can be seen. This is the theatre of self.

As she comes closer I *really* see her. We are in the same space. The heroine is center stage. We meet in the now; I am truly present with her. I hear her voice—the tone, the feeling, the quality, the energy behind the words. I see her physical self—how she moves, her gestures, her tiny micromovements. Almost always in the beginning there is something about the person that jumps out at me, out of the background into the foreground. It is a key that opens the treasure chest of mystery, the secret self, the core of the person. A key that reveals the divine spirit, the dæmon within.

The heroine lies down on her back on the soft surface of the massage table. My ego must get out of the way so that I may be present for her story. Silently I say a prayer that I may be totally available to the healing energy that will come through me.

We meet in a new way as I bring the palms of my hands very slowly toward her head. I feel her energy long before I am in physical contact. When I touch her head, it is no ordinary touch. It is oh so gentle, like a butterfly landing on a delicate blossom. I cradle her head. Men and women alike often tell me, with tears in their eyes, that to be touched with such care is rare in their lives.

I follow the energy in her body with my listening hands. They move with the changes in her energy. The drama begins—high play. I follow the heroine's process like a Greek chorus: repeating, reflecting, offering possibilities for change. The experience of the heroine becomes the experience of the group, the healing community surrounding the "altar." Her story can be like a soft rain, which, nourishing the soul, nourishes the group, too. Or it can be a series of fast-moving thunderstorms with lightning and immediate thunder that strike close to home. The waves of energy roll out from the table and engulf the group. And then the compassion and healing energy of the group return to the table to support the next wave.

The community is a healing circle. This is not entertainment. Her story is our story. She sings the song of herself, the body electric. This is the whole world as a stage, the divine comedy in all its forms, as I support with touch and with words the freeing of the genie held in this personal bottle. We laugh, with the heroine, at the absurdities of existence, and we cry with her sadnesses. As the heroine is freed of her torments, a catharsis sweeps through the community. We feel lighter, freed of some of our own feelings, touched by the universal themes that have been revealed.

When her story is finished, the heroine gets up from the table. She radiates her own personal energy. Her transformation is obvious to everyone who sees her. Her universal themes have touched many. As she returns to the community, she is appreciated and applauded. I feel ecstatic, full of energy, grateful to have supported the re-creation of wholeness in the heroine.

Is this magic? No. This resurrection of the spirit, emotions, body, and mind does not happen only at conferences. I have often experienced this transformation as an audience of one in my private practice. It may be repeated hundreds of times a day wherever Rubenfeld Synergists meet clients. We have all learned this "healing theatre" through Rubenfeld Synergy Training Programs. It takes time, but anyone who truly wants to do healing work in the world is a candidate to become a Rubenfeld Synergist.

Acknowledgments

I wish to thank those who made this book possible, especially:

My fellow Synergists Suzanne Forman, Jeanne Reock, Linda Thomas, and Alreta Turner, without whose early encouragement I would not have undertaken *Healing Journeys* and without whose continued support I might not have persevered.

Ilana Rubenfeld, my teacher, who warned me of many pitfalls, patiently answered countless historical questions, and referred me to people with interesting Synergy stories to tell.

The seventy-two Synergists and former Synergy clients who submitted proposals, stories, essays, poems, and works of art.

The contributing authors who trusted me with their stories and eagerly participated in seemingly endless rounds of revision— or patiently tolerated them—in order to communicate the power and subtleties of the Rubenfeld Synergy Method.

The scores of Synergists and trainees whose enthusiasm and expressions of appreciation cheered me on.

Readers who had no experience of Rubenfeld Synergy before reading drafts of these stories, who pointed out what worked and what didn't: Lisa Berger, Leo Braudy, Ronnie Bramesco, Johanna Cooper, Lillian Cozzarelli, Daniel Dearyan, John C. Driscoll, Leann Fecho, Gary Floam, Judy Floam, Stella Forster, Laura Fries, Gino Giglio, Vicki Gleicher, Edie Hartmann, Svend Hartmann, David Helman, David Janeway, Laurilyn D. Jones, Janine Jordan, Dana Keeler, Barbara Kovach, Peter Lillie, David A. Mechner, Emily Mechner, Francis Mechner, Jordan Mechner, Ashley Miller, Margaret Miller, Kristin Onofrio, Linda Partida, Herb Reynolds, Ilse Rosenberg, Norma Rosenberg, Bruce Rosenbloom, Harris Schiller, Laura Schiller, Sara Smith, Joe Sucher, Suzanne Sykes, Abe Weitzberg, Mary Weitzberg, Oscar C. Weitzberg.

Readers with direct experience of Rubenfeld Synergy, whose sensitive comments and suggestions led to further refinements: Ellen Blaney, Millison Farr Brace, Katherine Cates, Erin Colligan, Shirley Norwood, Linda Osmer, Claudine Paris, Jane Parsons-Fein, Margaret A. Healy, Irv Katz, Ronni B. Silett, Erica Sucher, Billie Thompson, Barb Weitzberg, Jeffrey K. Zeig; Master Synergists Elaine Burns Chapline, Millie Grenough, Florence Korzinski, Peggy Shaw Rosato, Joe Weldon, Noël Wight.

Linda Thomas—for coaching me on the ethical aspects of publishing stories by or about former clients. Kenneth G. Page — for the subtitle. Laura Jorstad, Ed Klagsbrun, Cindy LaBreacht, Sharon Lee Ryder, and Karyn Slutsky—for their artistic and technical skills and their guidance in navigating the complex world of book publishing.

About the Authors

Carol Smith Ali is a Certified Rubenfeld Synergist who has maintained a private practice in Asheville, North Carolina, since 1995. She completed the three-year Rubenfeld Synergy Post-graduate Training in 1997. Carol has also trained in Rogerian and Jungian therapy, Gestalt practice, and dreamwork. As a volunteer, she gives in-service trainings for hospice staff about the use of touch. Her hobbies include writing, music, modern dance, hiking, and pursuing her interest in holistic health.

Patti Allen has a rich and varied background in the healing arts, education, management and public speaking. Certified as a Rubenfeld Synergist, Patti runs a private practice in Toronto, Canada, and serves on the teaching staff of the Rubenfeld Synergy

Method Training Program—its twelfth training, (New York City 1994–1997) and its fifteenth (Toronto 1998–2002). Patti also facilitates dreamgroups, in which participants are assisted in understanding themselves through their dreams, both with and without the use of touch. Patti is cofounder, along with teacher, friend, colleague and "flying partner" Marjorie Paleshi, of Pathways to Healing, Inc.

Rose Andrzejewski has finally found her professional niche! Since completing the Rubenfeld Synergy Method Training Program she has been developing her private practice of Rubenfeld Synergy in Manhattan, where she especially enjoys working with clients who have difficulty finding their true vocation. Rose is also developing her cabaret act in Manhattan and will begin performing it in the fall of 1999.

Valerie Bain is a registered nurse in London, Ontario (Canada), where she has maintained her independent practice, "Wellness Services," for over ten years. She is certified in Rubenfeld Synergy, Reflexology, and Therapeutic Touch. A cancer survivor for over fourteen years despite two recurrences, Valerie counts among her clients many persons dealing with the physical, mental and emotional aspects of this disease. Valerie cosponsors two holistic health fairs in London annually and has brought to London speakers such as Ilana Rubenfeld and Drs. Bernie Siegel and Deepak Chopra, who have strongly influenced her own personal healing journey.

Gail Benton has been practicing Rubenfeld Synergy in Tucson, Arizona, since her 1991 certification. Her areas of specialization include: recovery from physical and emotional trauma; the building of wellness and self-esteem; and transforming grief, loss, conflict, pain, and stress into joyful living. Gail has been a mental health practitioner for twenty-five years. She is currently incorporating Rubenfeld Synergy into her work with hospice patients and their families. Gail is a longtime student and teacher of yoga and is an avid swimmer. She has two daughters, aged sixteen and eleven.

Marita Bishop began her quest for integrating body, mind, and soul at age thirty-six, when her esophagus "shut down." After medical science relieved her acute symptoms, Marita began exploring the contributing emotional, mental, and spiritual blocks. As a massage practitioner, she already knew the healing power of touch. Now as a Rubenfeld Synergist practicing in Snohomish, Washington, Marita finds that "our bodies are windows through which we learn to see and accept ourselves. Our wounds become building blocks in our healing." Marita's experience as a teacher and as mother of five serves her well in facilitating others' healing journeys.

Thomas Claire was enjoying the fruits of a successful career in finance when, in his late thirties, he began a search for deeper values. After exploring various metaphysical traditions and a variety of bodywork and body–mind therapies, he left the financial world to build a professional practice in bodywork and to research and write *Bodywork,* a guide to sixteen major body–mind methods. He continues to explore his interest in the full spectrum of mind–body practices through teaching, writing, and facilitating personal transformation.

Sonja Contois has been interested in philosophy, psychology, religion, and the spirit since her early teens. Those interests became passions, and at fifty-nine the passion remains. Because of Sonja's life goals and strong belief in the spirit of community, she dedicates one-third of her practice in Asheville, North Carolina, to pro bono work with breast cancer patients. Describing her work Sonja has said, "I experience my practice in Rubenfeld Synergy Method as something between a ministry, applied philosophy, and chiropractic for the soul. I cannot imagine another professional endeavor that would bring forth so much of an understanding of life."

Bernard Coyne is a member of the Council of Master Synergists. He teaches the Workshop Group Leadership Training with Ilana Rubenfeld and gives workshop presentations nationally and internationally. He is the cofounder—with his wife Dorothy Ann —of Sunnyside, a learning center in the Irish Hills of Michigan near Ann Arbor. There he has his private practice in Rubenfeld Synergy and teaches "Your Creative Process."

Patricia Ellen practices Rubenfeld Synergy in Scarsdale and Nyack, New York. In addition she draws on her background as an Interfaith minister, hypnotherapist, breathworker, and even as a certified public accountant. Patricia believes that times of transition and loss present individuals with a unique opportunity to transform the "tomb of loss" into the "womb of new ways of being." While integrating the pragmatic with the psychological and spiritual, she gently empowers her clients to create the lives, relationships, health, and financial well-being they desire. She says, "God danced the day you were born; now find your special dance. L'Chayim."

Betty Esthelle began her hands-on healing work in 1945, as a nurse. By 1977, when she began her training in the Rubenfeld Synergy Method, Betty's focus had changed from traditional medicine to esoteric healing. Since 1979 she has maintained her home and private practice, "Body Enlightenment," in San Francisco. The year 1984 was transformational—with Betty's divorce, near-death, cancer, and spontaneous healing. Betty has taught at the Gestalt Institute in Germany every year since 1985. She now travels extensively to teach the professional training program she has developed.

Lydia Foerster is an independent videomaker living in New York City. When she's not traveling the world for corporate clients, Lydia teaches video production at New York University and produces her own documentaries. Of all the stories she has lensed, none have been as intense or dramatic as the tales told on a table at 115 Waverly Place in Greenwich Village. After a year of shooting Rubenfeld Synergy sessions, Lydia volunteered for a "hip release." She promptly found her own Synergist, whom she has been seeing once a week ever since.

Suzanne Forman is a Certified Rubenfeld Synergist practicing in Northampton, Massachusetts. She is licensed as a massage therapist and also brings to her Rubenfeld Synergy practice years of study in yoga, CranioSacral Therapy, Gestalt Therapy, and Body–Mind Centering. Suzanne lives with her husband, Steve Forman, also a Certified Rubenfeld Synergist, and their daughter. She is on the board of directors of the National Association of Rubenfeld Synergists and is the founder of a holistic group practice in Northampton.

Joy Gates is a writer, artist, and eclectic adventurer in consciousness. She has lived in other countries, been married several times, raised three daughters, been a Tarot reader, astrologer and palmist, ranch caretaker, assistant manager of a health food store, and assistant director of an esoteric correspondence school. Her most grounded and practical work was accomplished on the bodywork table at Lalitha Devi's Manhattan office, where she was a Rubenfeld Synergy client twice a month for almost three years.

Suzanne Gluck-Sosis gives Rubenfeld Synergy much of the credit for her growth and transformation. Says Suzanne, "Previously a fearful and depressed widow with a deep sense of unworthiness, I have blossomed into a vibrant, energetic therapist, wife, and grandmother. This gentle, nonintrusive process created a safe place for exploring all facets of me—the light as well as the shadow—and to know that all of me is lovable." Recently remarried after twenty-one years of widowhood, Suzanne has relocated to Greenfield, Massachusetts, to be near her children and grandchildren and to continue her practice of Rubenfeld Synergy.

Erica Goodstone received her doctorate in human sexuality from New York University. On the faculty of the American Academy of Clinical Sexologists and a Professor of Health and Physical Education, she is also licensed as a mental health counselor, marriage counselor, and massage therapist and is certified as a Rubenfeld Synergist, Registered Polarity Practitioner, Oriental Bodywork Therapist, and Sex Counselor and Therapist. Dr. Goodstone divides her time between teaching, writing, and her private practice, which is basically Rubenfeld Synergy with a special focus on sexual and relationship issues.

Suzanne Selby Grenager lives and writes on a central Pennsylvania farm. She is certified in both the Rubenfeld Synergy Method and Kripalu Yoga, and has shared yoga with thousands of people. As Kripalu's longtime Mid-Atlantic Regional Leader, Sue supported group leaders in helping others grow through yoga and, in 1994, received Kripalu's Global Service Award for exemplary leadership and service. A former *Philadelphia Inquirer* columnist,

Sue writes articles and is working on a book, *Relax, Trust, Love: How To Be Powerfully Human and Like It, at Least Sometimes.* She and her husband, Trond, have two grown children.

Millie Grenough was in Ilana's second Rubenfeld Synergy Training and is a member of the Council of Master Synergists. Her five years' experience working with varied cultures in Latin America and Europe piqued her interest in the connections between body, mind and spirit. Millie has a Master of Arts degree in teaching, is a licensed clinical social worker, and is the author of *Sing It! Learn English Through Song* (McGraw-Hill). A professional singer, she has a special interest in helping people find their body–voice connection and in teaching stress management and self-care to business groups and individuals.

Margaret A. Healy is a Certified Rubenfeld Synergist who came to train in the method after learning, from her experience with modern dance and choreography, the importance of listening to the body. She has eighteen years' experience working with infants and young children, and is continually awed by their vitality and freedom of movement. Margaret hopes to practice Rubenfeld Synergy with children, helping them restore their innate love of their bodies by increasing their awareness of the external messages that have led to their unnatural and restrictive holding patterns. Margaret practices in Morristown, New Jersey, and New York City.

Estela M. Hernandez is an educator and health care practitioner on a journey of exploration. Dedicated to serving humanity, she has been seeking a higher truth in the field of health care. Trained as a research nurse-biologist, she lives and works in Queens, New York, where she maintains a Rubenfeld Synergy practice and teaches human biology for the City University of New York. She is currently researching and developing for her college a curriculum in holistic health care. As a workshop leader she is dedicated to introducing the Rubenfeld Synergy Method to her students and the people in her community.

Mary Jane Hooper practices at the Wellness Center in Fort Worth, Texas, a center dedicated to promoting health and preventing illness. Mary Jane has a master's degree in marriage and family therapy from Texas Woman's University and has trained in several integrative approaches to working with individuals, couples, and families. By encouraging her Rubenfeld Synergy clients to explore the wisdom of the body, Mary Jane finds that they are often able to free their perceptions, rewrite their life stories, and nurture forgotten strengths. Mary Jane enjoys life with her husband, Win, and their two cats and chihuahua puppy.

Mary Hopkins, age forty-two, is a classically trained singer and professional musician living in New England. She performs in a range of musical genres and styles, and works as a choral conductor, voice teacher, composer, and arranger. Mary uses the insights gained through Rubenfeld Synergy along with extensive formal training in music to enrich all her musical endeavors. She particularly enjoys working with students who are striving to overcome obstacles to their singing and performing. Mary's other interests include gardening, herbalism, and living thankfully.

Diane Junglas's desire to support and guide others in reaching their potential laid the foundation for her doctoral research exploring the integrative experience of Rubenfeld Synergy. As a clinician she nurtures others' healing and growth through creatively blending her knowledge and skills in psychology, Rubenfeld Synergy, and Polarity Therapy. Diane has worked with adults, groups, and couples for twenty years. A cocreator of the Life Resonance Center, a healing and educational center in the metropolitan Detroit area, she teaches skills in the therapeutic use of the self to health care professionals and is available for presentations and consultations.

Peggy Kostyshyn practices Rubenfeld Synergy in Thunder Bay, Ontario. She brings to this work thirty years of nursing experience, many years as an active hockey/ballet/scouting mom, and a lifetime of volunteer work starting in eighth grade, when she organized Thunder Bay's first Alateen group. Says Peggy, "Everything I did before Rubenfeld Synergy was out of my need to correct feelings of inadequacy from my past. Now I do everything out of love of life. What I want to share with my clients is the happiness and joy that are waiting for us all."

Greg Kowalski lived and trained in Japan with Dr. Masaaki Hatsumi, the current Grandmaster of the Ninja, and is one of the world's seniormost instructors of Ninjutsu. In addition to his ninth-degree black belt in Ninjutsu, which he teaches throughout the country, Greg holds rank in several other martial arts. He maintains his school (New England Ninjutsu) and his Rubenfeld Synergy practice in Wallingford, Connecticut. A serious outdoorsman and camper, Greg has trained with Tom Brown in primitive living skills and nature awareness and is interested in Native American spirituality.

Margaret Cappi Lang is director of the Prescott Center for the Arts in Healing and the Practice of Rubenfeld Synergy. She maintains her practice in Prescott and Phoenix, Arizona. She received a master's degree from Pratt Institute (New York) in the expressive therapies and a doctorate in human development from Arizona State University. She is a certified supervisor for both art therapy and Rubenfeld Synergy and currently teaches art therapy at Prescott College. A practicing artist, Cappi also enjoys singing and dancing. Cappi's fiancé, Bill, is building a studio in which Cappi hopes to establish a retreat space for the Center.

Lee McAvoy is a writer, teacher, and Certified Rubenfeld Synergist practicing in Rochester, New York. She also works with pets, using a system she developed called "Harjo Animal Touch," which combines elements of Rubenfeld Synergy, Reiki, and Therapeutic Touch.

Annie McCaffry has studied parapsychology for the past thirty-five years, focusing on inherited family patterns that result in disease. She is a practicing consultant and conference speaker. In 1993 her *Journey to My Self* was published by Element Books of Shaftesbury, England. Annie is at present engaged in a follow-up book on the power of light and sound in healing and a television series centered around some of the challenges facing us in the next century. She lives and maintains a practice in Ramsbury, Wiltshire, England.

Barbara McKenzie's introduction to the connection between body, mind, and spirit came through her twenty-year study and teaching of the philosophy and discipline of Hatha Yoga. Her health and sense of well-being improved with her practice of yoga and her studies of the principles of metaphysics. Her creative expression, in the form of writing poetry, increased along with her spiritual development. Barbara recognized Rubenfeld Synergy as her ultimate calling when she attended a workshop given by Ilana. Barbara is currently a second-year student in the four-year Rubenfeld Synergy Training Program.

Gay Marcontell was an artist before training to be a Rubenfeld Synergist. She worked in mixed media—paint, pencil, clay, autumn leaves—anything, in short, she could get her hands on. She has a bachelor of fine arts degree with work in oils and print-making. She has practiced and taught journaling and meditation for many years. To expand her skills as a Synergist, group leader, supervisor, and teacher of Rubenfeld Synergy Method, Gay is serving as a teaching intern with the current Rubenfeld Synergy training class.

P. Tanzy Maxfield lives with her partner, Rolf Godon, Ph.D., on the Truckee River in Truckee, California, thirty miles west of Reno, Nevada. At their professional center, Water by the River, Rolf practices psychotherapy and Tanzy practices Rubenfeld Synergy and Hellerwork. Certified by Harville Hendrix, together they produce "Getting the Love You Want" couples' workshops. Between them they have four marriages, four divorces, four children, and two grandchildren. In their fifteen years together, they have even survived the building of their house. Says Tanzy, "We practice in our lives and our relationship what we teach."

Vicki Mechner found Rubenfeld Synergy in the early nineties after an eighteen-month search for a body–mind method that would help her keep loved ones out of hospitals. Upon her certification as a Rubenfeld Synergist, she thought she had left behind previous careers in editing, educational design, matchmaking, and marketing—but everything she ever knew came in handy in producing *Healing Journeys*. Vicki practices Rubenfeld Synergy and Bowen Technique in New York City and Chappaqua, New York, and enjoys helping people maximize their well-being and effectiveness. She and her husband of thirty-seven years have four grown children.

Bill Miller first met Ilana Rubenfeld over twenty years ago, when he photographed her workshops. At the time, he was part of the spiritual community known as Pathwork. Bill has been a recognized Pathwork Helper (therapist) and group leader since 1985 and has trained in Core Energetics. While achieving success as a photographer, he realized that if money were not an issue, he would devote his life to working with people on a very deep psychological and physical level to foster transformation; he thus trained to become a Certified Rubenfeld Synergist. He now balances photography and Synergy.

Diane Montgomery-Logan has been exploring the human psyche since 1986, when she decided to leave a career as a metalsmith to become a psychotherapist. Seven years later she saw Rubenfeld Synergy as the opportunity to again use her hands in creative work. Her passion is for the spiritual dimension of her practice, the opportunity to accompany clients in their search for themselves. She lives in Burlington, Vermont, where she loves to garden in the summer and dance the fox-trot the rest of the year. Diane chairs the Ethics Committee and serves on the board of directors of the National Association of Rubenfeld Synergists.

Meg Morris practices Rubenfeld Synergy in Cincinnati, Ohio, where by day she is a technical sales professional in the telecommunications industry. She attributes her success in that industry to her ability to listen and hear her customers' needs. Once less active, Meg now works out five days each week, plays volleyball frequently, coaches two girls' volleyball teams, and has recently begun long-distance bicycling. Meg attributes her high energy and good humor to lots of personal work and the loving influences of her boyfriend, Paul, and their blended family of five dogs, one cat, and fifteen tanks of freshwater fish.

Renate M. Novak was born to a single mother in Germany in 1950. Renate moved to the United States in 1970 just after graduating from a two-and-a-half-year full-time training at a holistic health school. Since then, she has been working as a massage therapist. Her primary focus since 1991 has been as the owner and codirector of Health Choices, a holistic massage therapy school near Princeton, New Jersey. Most of Renate's personal healing work has been accomplished through body-centered psychotherapies, including Rubenfeld Synergy.

Bineke Oort is a Rubenfeld Synergist and a Licensed Family Therapist. Having been sensitized to the effects of trauma through her own experiences, Bineke has a particular affinity for clients recovering from trauma. Bineke is also a storyteller specializing in sacred stories. She currently serves on the board of directors of the National Association of Rubenfeld Synergists. Bineke and her husband, Abraham, who practice Mindful Meditation as taught by Thich Nhat Hanh, realize more and more that paradise can be found here on Earth. Bineke has a master's degree in social work and a private practice in Rubenfeld Synergy.

Jeanne Reock is a Certified Rubenfeld Synergist practicing in the Princeton, New Jersey, area since 1991. She is president of both the National Association of Rubenfeld Synergists and the Holistic Health Association of the Princeton Area (HHAPA). After a long career working to influence state policy regarding public education, Jeanne takes great pleasure in helping people grow into their true essence, person by person. Her approach to therapy is simply a further reflection of her passion for educating the "whole person—body, mind, and soul" in a way that honors each individual's unique being.

Toni Luisa Rivera, a Certified Rubenfeld Synergist and doctor of chiropractic, practices full-time in Santa Fe, New Mexico. Toni is also on the staff of the Rubenfeld Synergy

Training. Her hobbies range from riding horseback to riding the waves of the ocean when she visits her native island of Puerto Rico.

Gisèle Robert is a registered nurse who trained in Gestalt Therapy, Therapeutic Touch, visualization, and Jungian dream analysis before entering the Rubenfeld Synergy Training Program. Gisèle has earned a degree in psychosociology and master's degrees in personal communication and psychology. She has founded an association of nurses offering alternative care in Québec and has taught at universities and trained many caretakers in hospice care. Currently on the board of directors of the Québec Gestalt Association, she offers workshops on self-care and on dream body-mapping. Gisèle's private practice as a Rubenfeld Synergist is in Montréal.

Mike Schlesinger is a licensed psychologist who lives near Philadelphia in Ambler, Pennsylvania. He grew up in Forest Hills, New York, went to Case Western Reserve in Cleveland, and received a doctorate in psychoeducational processes from Temple University. In his private practice Dr. Schlesinger sees individuals, couples, and families. As word of body-oriented psychotherapy continues to spread, more and more of his clients are choosing to use the Rubenfeld Synergy Method instead of traditional psychotherapy. Mike and his wife, also a psychotherapist, enjoy skiing, biking, and traveling with their teenage son and daughter.

Carol Seewald is a body-centered practitioner and Certified Rubenfeld Synergist. Carol worked as a counselor and administrator for La Leche League Canada for fifteen years, as a speech and language pathologist for fourteen, and a Therapeutic Touch practitioner for thirteen. Her personal roles as partner with her husband of twenty-eight years and mother of three have provided fertile ground for learning to live in peaceful, passionate, and safe community in this swiftly changing world. Currently she has a private practice in London, Ontario.

Linda Stoffel brings to her work as a Rubenfeld Synergist and massage therapy practitioner knowledge acquired through a lifetime of travel, work, and play. In her work as a somatic educator, she draws upon her career as office manager and secretary and her more recent vocation as a wall-hanging designer, and also incorporates her gifts as folk singer–guitarist, landscape gardener, weaver, and outdoorswoman. Since her certification in 1994, Ms. Stoffel has practiced Rubenfeld Synergy—first in Harper's Ferry, West Virginia, and now in Dora, Missouri, where she provides a holistic healing experience.

Gilly Thomas was inspired to write when, after her first week of Rubenfeld Synergy Training, her dead marriage came back to life. Now a happy stay-at-home mum to her four-year-old daughter, Tekarra, Gilly spends her "free" time skiing, running, and hiking in the Canadian Rockies and training in Rubenfeld Synergy, preparing for certification in the year 2000. Gilly writes: "I always sensed that there was more to people than the verbal rationalizations they put forth in the world. I also realized that there was more to me than what I put forth to myself and others."

Linda Thomas has been a practicing therapist for eighteen years, helping families heal and helping individuals find their home in their hearts. She has worked extensively with families and individuals experiencing severe crises and despair. She seeks to create a balance in her work by bringing her belief in love, humor, and basic human goodness into her sessions. Rubenfeld Synergy has been her model for attaining this harmony, following an education and training in philosophy, ethics, clinical social work, and archetypal psychology. She was the first Ethics Committee Chair of the National Association of Rubenfeld Synergists. She practices in Wickford and Newport, Rhode Island.

Donna L. Ulanowski, a licensed clinical professional counselor and Certified Rubenfeld Synergist, established the Personal Growth Centre in Olympia Fields, Illinois. In addition to practicing Rubenfeld Synergy there, she conducts workshops and in-service training programs in team-building, communication, stress management, enhancing creativity and productivity in the workplace, the mind–body connection, and self-care for the caregiver. Donna loves canoeing and kayaking and has taught tai chi for several years. Donna is a teaching intern in the current Rubenfeld Synergy Training class.

Paul Valiulis lives and works in the mountains but is a water person at heart. A mountain guide trained and certified by the Association of Canadian Mountain Guides, Paul teaches people how to climb mountains, rocks, and ice, as well as ski in the backcountry. When not in the hills Paul enjoys spending time with his family, taking pictures, and swimming.

A Brief History
of Rubenfeld Synergy

As a teenager Ilana Rubenfeld was surrounded by music at home and at school. She played several instruments—viola, flute, oboe, and piano—but her passion was conducting. In the mid-fifties, after auditioning for and being accepted into the conducting program at the Juilliard School of Music, she was well on her way toward her goal when a debilitating back spasm changed the course of her life.

Seeking help, she discovered Judith Leibowitz, a teacher of the F. M. Alexander Technique, which uses gentle touch to educate the bodymind and help muscles relax. She taught Ilana how to use her body more efficiently, thereby easing the tensions and spasms. Judy also taught her how to continue conducting without causing pain or reinjury.

But during these lessons Ilana began to experience early memories and express intense emotions. Judy did not know how to process these stories and outbursts of feelings. She subsequently referred Ilana to a psychoanalyst, who asked Ilana to recall the memories and express the emotions that sometimes emerged when she was on the Alexander table. Although she could describe them, Ilana could not reexperience the feelings that had been evoked by the Alexander touch. As the analyst continued to analyze events in her life, Ilana asked him to consider using touch, too. He recoiled at the suggestion.

Ilana worked with both professionals for several years, gaining important experiences and insights from each. As she came to realize that the analysis and the bodywork were equally important, she yearned to have one professional use both modalities simultaneously so that she could more easily connect and integrate what she was learning from them separately.

She continued to study the Alexander Technique and became a certified teacher. While working with many students, Ilana observed that a vital element was missing for them as it was for her: a way to process the emotional material that was locked in the body. She longed to know her clients' emotional history, stresses, and life problems, which had created their physical dysfunctions in the first place.

Soon after, she conceived a method that combined bodywork, touch, and psychotherapy. Then the hard work began: researching, studying, and experimenting. Her curiosity and studies led her to train and collaborate with Dr. Peter Hogan, an Adlerian psychiatrist, Drs. Fritz and Laura Perls, cofounders of Gestalt Therapy, and Moshe Feldenkrais, founder of the Feldenkrais Method. Inspired by these studies she continuously refined the integration of bodywork and psychotherapy.

By the early seventies, in addition to teaching the Alexander

Technique and Gestalt Therapy, Ilana maintained a full private practice using her own eclectic approach—integrating movement, gentle touch, verbal expression, imagery, and a large dose of humor. She discovered that trust and strong therapeutic relationships flourished when sessions took place in an environment of safety and nonjudgment.

The therapeutic results were so impressive that by 1975, in response to increasing demand for Rubenfeld Synergy, Ilana began to develop a pedagogic approach and curriculum for a professional certification training program. Between the first class (1977–1979) and the fifteenth class (1998–2002), the Rubenfeld Synergy Training Program has been refined and expanded to its current four-year, sixteen hundred-hour format.

Ilana says, "The first step to client care is self-care." Accordingly, an important component of the training program is learning to practice self-care while giving sessions. In addition to the lectures, demonstrations, discussions, supervised practice, body-mind exercises, and individual projects, the training includes a great deal of humor, tears, and laughter.

Coming from a strong musical background, Ilana developed a process for annotating all the verbal and nonverbal events that occur at each moment of a Rubenfeld Synergy session, as well as the significance of what is happening. The process is similar to the one Ilana had learned at Juilliard for analyzing musical scores. Trainees develop their observational skills by studying and analyzing a videotaped session and "scoring" it using this process.

To enable trainees to learn at their own pace and in their own style, individual attention and supervision and a high teacher-to-student ratio were required. Ilana developed a postgraduate program to train qualified Synergists to become faculty and provide continuity for each training class. The training community developed into an active culture for learning, growth, and support.

Ilana asked the training faculty to assist her in establishing a code of ethics to help guide trainees and Synergists in their professional dealings with clients. Some of the areas covered in this code are: respect and confidentiality; sensitivity to the difference in power between practitioners and clients; avoiding personal relationships; maintaining clear boundaries with clients. Before receiving certification, trainees are required to demonstrate an understanding of this code and sign an agreement to adhere to it.

To date (July 1998) Ilana and her faculty have certified over 350 Rubenfeld Synergists. After certification most Synergists continue their personal sessions and receive ongoing supervision; some undertake advanced professional training in Rubenfeld Synergy and related fields.

In 1994 Ilana formed the Council of Master Synergists by appointing nine Synergists[1] as charter members—all highly experienced in private practice and longtime members of the teaching staff. She invited them to present Rubenfeld Synergy workshops and to participate with her as colleagues in making policy. The Council's mission statement is "to embody, express, and creatively teach the healing power of the Rubenfeld Synergy Method to the community at large."

A group of certified Synergists living in Canada formed a professional association in 1994. A year later, Ilana invited a group of certified Synergists to do the same in the United States. (See "Resources," page 337.)

At these associations' annual conferences, Synergists share their experiences in using Rubenfeld Synergy with couples, families, business organizations, and individuals suffering from eating dis-

---

[1] Rob Bauer, Elaine Burns Chapline, Bernard Coyne, Millie Grenough, Florence Korzinski, Peggy Shaw Rosato, Judy Swallow, Joe Weldon, Noël Wight.

orders, brain injuries, performance anxiety, cancer, post-traumatic stress disorder, and terminal illnesses.

A Rubenfeld Synergy Session

A typical session lasts about forty-five minutes and can be conducted privately, in an ongoing group, or in the context of a workshop. At various times during the session, the client may lie down, sit, stand, and move around. Synergist and client(s) remain fully clothed at all times.

Clients are in charge of their sessions' pace and direction, and may stop a session at any time for any reason. No diagnoses are made, nor cures promised. Sessions usually begin with current or recent events in clients' lives, then may move to past events and/or to the future. When appropriate, Synergists use their listening touch to hear the body's story simultaneously with the verbal story.

Although Rubenfeld Synergy may bring life-changing insights in a short time, weekly sessions for at least several months to years are suggested for fully integrated and lasting benefits.

Rubenfeld Synergy BodyMind Exercises

Inspired by Moshe Feldenkrais's work, Ilana integrated a great deal of imagery and metaphor into bodymind exercises. These exercises not only ease tensions, foster flexibility, develop coordination, and teach "inner awareness," but may also support the melting of tight emotional holding patterns in the body, encourage memories to emerge, and promote the expression of feelings.

Synergists often suggest specific bodymind exercises to their clients, who can practice them at home between sessions. During the training program, a different exercise is taught each day in order to increase trainees' awareness of their own body–mind interconnections and those of the clients they touch and move.

Benefits and Contraindications

Clients often report improvements in body image, clarity, sense of purpose, and relationships with family members and friends; relief from pain; increases in energy, range of motion, body awareness, self-esteem, and self-acceptance.

There are no known contraindications to receiving Rubenfeld Synergy sessions, nor are there dangerous side effects. Synergists are trained to recognize situations that need referral to other professionals.

Resources

For information about the Rubenfeld Synergy Method and the Rubenfeld Synergy Training Program, contact:

> The Rubenfeld Synergy Center
> 115 Waverly Place
> New York, NY 10011
> 1-800-747-6897
> e-mail: rubenfeld@aol.com
> http://members.aol.com/rubenfeld/synergy/index.html

For referrals to certified Rubenfeld Synergists, contact:

> National Association of Rubenfeld Synergists
> 1000 River Road, Suite 8H
> Belmar, NJ 07719 USA

National Association of Rubenfeld Synergists *(continued)*
1-800-484-3250, code 8516
e-mail: nars@home.com
www.rubenfeldsynergy.ca

Canadian Association of Rubenfeld Synergists
112 Lund Street
Richmond Hill, ONT L4C 5V9 CANADA
1-877-890-8484 or (905)883-3158
e-mail: alreta@ilap.com
www.rubenfeldsynergy.ca

Both of these associations seek to educate the public about the Rubenfeld Synergy Method, to foster members' professional development, and to protect the right of Synergists to practice. Each organization's code of ethics holds its members to high standards of professional ethics. Designed to protect clients and ensure professional integrity by upholding the standards, values, and practice of the Rubenfeld Synergy Method, the codes articulate ethical responsibilities to clients, colleagues, the profession, and the broader society.

Both professional associations provide copies of their code of ethics upon request.

Bibliography

Claire, T. (1995). Rubenfeld Synergy Method: Touch therapy meets talk therapy. In *Bodywork*. New York: William Morrow and Company, Inc., 151–165.

Forman, S. (1998). The Rubenfeld Synergy Method addresses mind, body and spirit. *Massage Magazine*, Issue 71, Jan./Feb., 70–80.*

Junglas, D. (1994). *The experience of becoming an integrated self through Rubenfeld Synergy*. Unpublished (doctoral dissertation, The Union Institute. Ann Arbor: University Microfilms Publishing).

Lerklin, J. M. (1995). Sing the body electric. *Changes*, June, 30–35.*

Markowitz, L. (1996). Minding the body, embodying the mind: Therapists explore mind-body alternatives. *Family Therapy Networker*, Sept.–Oct., 20–33. *

MetaMedia Arts. (1995). *Ilana Rubenfeld: Growing old means forgetting to retire*. Omega Institute, New Age Journal and MetaMedia Arts, A Time for Spirit Video Series from the Third Annual Conference on Conscious Aging.*

McCaffry, A. (1993). *Journey to my self: The healing of relationships & the transformation of family patterns*. Shaftesbury, England: Element Books. Available from the author at Chapel-on-the-Water, Ramsbury, Wiltshire SN8 2QN, UK. T/F: (44) 16725 20701.

Rubenfeld, I. (1972). Alexander technique and innovations. In American Dance Therapy Association, *Dance therapy: Roots and extensions.* Columbia MD: ADTA.

———. (1973). *Rubenfeld on the road.* (audiotapes). New York: The Rubenfeld Center, Inc.*

———. (1985). Self-care for the professional woman: Beyond physical fitness. In L. Knezek, M. Barrett, and S. Collins (eds.), *Women and work.* Arlington: University of Texas.

———. (1988). Beginner's hands: Twenty-five years of simple, Rubenfeld Synergy — the birth of a therapy. *Somatics,* vol. VI, no. 4, 4–11.*

———. (1990–91). Ushering in a century of integration. *Somatics,* vol. VIII, no. 1, 59–63.*

———. (1992). Gestalt therapy and the bodymind: an overview of the Rubenfeld Synergy® Method. In Edwin C. Nevis (ed.), *Gestalt therapy: Perspectives and applications.* New York: Gardner Press, Inc., 147–177.

———. (1992). *Ilana Rubenfeld: Mind-body integration, an InnerWork videotape with Dr. Jeffrey Mishlove.* Berkeley, CA: Thinking Allowed Productions.*

———. (1997). Healing the emotional/spiritual body. In Christine Caldwell (ed.), *Getting in touch: The guide to new body-centered therapies.* Wheaton, IL: Quest Books, 179–210.

———. (1998). The Rubenfeld Synergy Method. In Lynette Bassman (ed.), *The whole mind: The definitive guide to complementary treatments for mind, mood, and emotion.* Novato, CA: New World Library, 464–475.

Simon, R. (1997). Listening hands. *Family Therapy Networker,* Sept.–Oct., vol. XXI, no. 5, 62–73. *

1 Asterisks here indicate availability, from the Rubenfeld Synergy Center, of articles, reprints, audiotapes, and videotape cassettes.

Glossary and Guide to Pronunciation

ALEXANDER TECHNIQUE
Created by F. M. Alexander in the 1890s, this bodymind system employs gentle touch and specific verbal instructions to reeducate people about relaxing, moving, and improving their posture in everyday life. Although Alexander students may experience attitudinal and emotional changes as a result of their lessons, this approach does not directly address these emotional issues. After training with Judith Liebowitz, Ilana Rubenfeld taught the Alexander Technique for many years.

BODYMIND (noun)
The whole self, including both body and mind as an inseparable unit. (See also "soma" on page 345.) Physical sensations often influence our thoughts and emotions. The reverse is also true.

BODY-MIND (adjective)

As in "body–mind connection," this term emphasizes the relationship between body and mind, which for the last few centuries have frequently been thought of as separate entities. "Mind–body" means the same.

CENTERING; TO CENTER

The act of consciously bringing one's attention to oneself in order to become calm and available to what is happening in the present moment. Meditation is one method of centering. Feeling centered is the opposite of feeling scattered.

CERTIFIED RUBENFELD SYNERGIST (CRS)

(ROO-ben-fehld SINN-er-jist). The title used exclusively by practitioners who have fulfilled all the requirements of the Rubenfeld Synergy Training Program and have been certified by the training program and Ilana Rubenfeld.

CLIENT

A person who receives Rubenfeld Synergy sessions. See the introduction for reasons for saying "client" instead of "patient."

CRADLING; TO CRADLE

The act of gently holding and supporting the client's head, leg, or arm with open hands.

EMBODY

To demonstrate new beliefs and attitudes through unconscious changes in the body—breathing, posture, gesture, facial expression—rather than merely to hold the beliefs intellectually.

ERICKSONIAN HYPNOTHERAPY

In the 1930s psychiatrist Milton Erickson demystified hypnosis, defining it as highly focused attention and unconscious learning.

Erickson trusted the ability of his patients' unconscious to bring about therapeutic change. After aligning with a patient's metaphor, Erickson talked to the unconscious experiential patterns and introduced hypnotic suggestions for reorganizing the patterns toward greater health. After Erickson's death in 1980, Ilana Rubenfeld refined her understanding of the hypnotic use of touch and talk by training with a pupil of his, Jane Parsons-Fein.

FELDENKRAIS METHOD
(FELD-n-krice). Developed by Moshe Feldenkrais in the 1950s, this method teaches students how to improve their movement and thinking beyond their habitual patterns. It does this by intentionally varying their sensorimotor activity, either in group Awareness Through Movement classes or in private lessons called Functional Integration. Although students experience mental and emotional changes through this approach, it does not directly address emotional issues. Ilana Rubenfeld was certified in 1977 by Feldenkrais after completing his first professional training program in the United States.

GESTALT THERAPY
(guh-SHTAHLT). Developed in the late 1940s by Drs. Frederick S. (Fritz) and Laura Perls, this psychotherapeutic approach emphasizes awareness of present events, immediate experience, and inter-relational contact. It strives not to be analytical or interpretive, but rather encourages clients to find their own meanings, set their own goals, and make their own choices in the process of recovering aspects of themselves that were disowned or lost during their growth and development. The Gestalt Therapist creates "here-and-now" experiences (also called "creative experiments") that involve thinking, sensing, and feeling. After studying with the Perlses, Ilana taught Gestalt Therapy for many years.

ILANA RUBENFELD
(ih-LAH-nah ROO-ben-fehld). The creator of the Rubenfeld Synergy Method and founder of the Rubenfeld Synergy Center. Often called "the grande dame of body–mind integration," she is invariably referred to as "Ilana" by those who know her.

INTEGRATE; INTEGRATION
To become integrated is to bring together into an internally harmonious state all aspects of the self—body, mind, emotions, and spirit. People who are "well integrated" are self-aware and self-accepting, and are sometimes said to "have it together." Integration is the process of achieving that state.

LISTENING TOUCH
A specifically trained touch that can sense and read "messages" expressed through the body.

MODALITY
A form of—or approach to—bodywork or psychotherapy.

NOODLING
Using the fingertips to gently palpate muscles and soft tissue at the base of the skull or along the spine. This type of touch invites clients to become more aware of tensions there and, possibly, to release them.

PRACTICE CLIENTS
The Rubenfeld Synergy term for the volunteers with whom trainees practice the method's techniques and philosophy. Practice clients pay no fee and may receive only a limited number of sessions from any given trainee.

RUBENFELD SYNERGY METHOD
(ROO-ben-fehld SINN-er-jee) The system of body-oriented psychotherapy and reeducation developed by Ilana Rubenfeld in the

1960s. It fosters inner awareness through the use of gentle touch, verbal expression, movement, and intuition.

SOMA

(SOH-mah) The entire living body as perceived subjectively from the inside. This ancient Greek term includes self-awareness of feelings, movements, and intentions—aspects of knowledge that are not available to objective observers.

SOMATIC

(soh-MATT-ic) Pertaining to the soma or bodymind. In Rubenfeld Synergy the specific techniques of touching and moving clients, so as to enhance their self-awareness, are called "somatic skills."

SUPERVISION

There are three kinds of supervision in Rubenfeld Synergy:

• During each training week and at regional meetings, teachers supervise small groups of trainees practicing the various skills of Rubenfeld Synergy. These supervisors support the trainees' practice of self-care and their understanding of the choices they make when working with clients.

• During and between training weeks, trainees consult with their individual training supervisor about sessions with practice clients.

• After certification, Synergists may consult with specially trained supervisors about situations and dynamics in their ongoing practices. These consultations are also called "supervision."

SYNERGIST

In this book, a Rubenfeld Synergist.

SYNERGY

• Dictionary definition: Combined action or operation such that the total effect is greater than the sum of the separate effects.

• After Buckminster Fuller saw Ilana Rubenfeld demonstrate her work in the 1970s, he suggested that she rename it "synergy" because it went beyond the mere integration of touch, movement, and talk.

• Although others use the word, when Rubenfeld Synergists say "Synergy," they mean Rubenfeld Synergy.

TABLE

A comfortably padded table, similar to a massage table but without the headrest, on which clients often lie during Rubenfeld Synergy sessions.

TRAINEE

A student in the Rubenfeld Synergy Training Program.

Index

Notes

Order Form

To order with a credit card, phone toll-free: **1-800-356-9315**.

To order by mail, complete this form and send it with your check or money order to OmniQuest Press (see address below).

Please ship _____ copy(ies) of *Healing Journeys: The Power of Rubenfeld Synergy* to the following address. I understand that I may return the book(s) for a full refund—for any reason, no questions asked.

PLEASE AFFIX ADDRESS LABEL OR PRINT CLEARLY

Name:_____

Address:_____
                            STREET OR P.O. BOX

_____
            CITY   STATE   ZIP

Daytime telephone: (_____)_____ (We will call you only if we need to clarify something about your order.)

QUANTITY	ITEM	PRICE EACH	TOTAL
	Healing Journeys	$14.95 (U.S.)	
SHIPPING: $4.00 for the first copy, $1.00 each additional copy.			
N.Y.S. ADDRESSES: add appropriate sales tax.			
❑ Check ❑ M.O. (payable to OmniQuest Press)		TOTAL:	

OMNIQUEST PRESS • P. O. BOX 15 • CHAPPAQUA, NY 10514

Order Form

To order with a credit card, phone toll-free: **1-800-356-9315**.

To order by mail, complete this form and send it with your check or money order to OmniQuest Press (see address below).

Please ship _____ copy(ies) of *Healing Journeys: The Power of Rubenfeld Synergy* to the following address. I understand that I may return the book(s) for a full refund—for any reason, no questions asked.

PLEASE AFFIX ADDRESS LABEL OR PRINT CLEARLY

Name:_____

Address:_____
STREET OR P.O. BOX

_____
CITY   STATE   ZIP

Daytime telephone: (_____)_____ (We will call you only if we need to clarify something about your order.)

QUANTITY	ITEM	PRICE EACH	TOTAL
	Healing Journeys	$14.95 (U.S.)	
SHIPPING: $4.00 for the first copy, $1.00 each additional copy.			
N.Y.S. ADDRESSES: add appropriate sales tax.			
❑ Check ❑ M.O. (payable to OmniQuest Press) TOTAL:			

OMNIQUEST PRESS • P. O. BOX 15 • CHAPPAQUA, NY 10514

Order Form

To order with a credit card, phone toll-free: **1-800-356-9315**.

To order by mail, complete this form and send it with your check or money order to OmniQuest Press (see address below).

Please ship _____ copy(ies) of *Healing Journeys: The Power of Rubenfeld Synergy* to the following address. I understand that I may return the book(s) for a full refund—for any reason, no questions asked.

PLEASE AFFIX ADDRESS LABEL OR PRINT CLEARLY

Name:_____

Address:_____
STREET OR P.O. BOX

_____
CITY   STATE   ZIP

Daytime telephone: (_____)_____ (We will call you only if we need to clarify something about your order.)

QUANTITY	ITEM	PRICE EACH	TOTAL
	Healing Journeys	$14.95 (U.S.)	
SHIPPING: $4.00 for the first copy, $1.00 each additional copy.			
N.Y.S. ADDRESSES: add appropriate sales tax.			
❑ Check ❑ M.O. (payable to OmniQuest Press) TOTAL:			

OMNIQUEST PRESS • P. O. BOX 15 • CHAPPAQUA, NY 10514